Eat to Beat Cancer

Eat to Beat Cancer

A Nutritional Guide with 40 Delicious Recipes

Dr Rosy Daniel
and Jane Sen

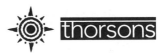

Thorsons
An Imprint of HarperCollins*Publishers*
77–85 Fulham Palace Road
Hammersmith, London W6 8JB

The website address is: www.thorsonselement.com

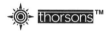

and *Thorsons* are trademarks of
HarperCollins*Publishers* Ltd

Published by Thorsons 2003
Many of the recipes in Chapter 5 have previously appeared in
Healing Foods Cookbook and *More Healing Foods* by Jane Sen

10 9 8 7

A catalogue record for this book is
available from the British Library

ISBN-13 978-0-00-714704-5
ISBN-10 0-00-714704-X

Printed and bound in Great Britain by
Martins the Printers Limited, Berwick upon Tweed

Dedication

Dr Rosy Daniel and Jane Sen would like to dedicate this book to those doctors and nutritionists who were initially ridiculed for pointing out the vital relationship between cancer and diet in the 1960s and 70s. Among those who led the way were Gerson, Issels, de Vries, Moerman, Kelly, Breuss, Contreras and Forbes. All of these doctors were deemed in their time to be irresponsible for suggesting that raw vegetables, fruits and whole foods contain the key elements to protect us from cancer. Now, 40 years later, the science has caught up with these pioneers and the main theme of all cancer-prevention programmes worldwide revolves around eating increased amounts of fruits and vegetables and a healthy non-processed diet. We honour them for their brilliance and bravery in withstanding so much criticism and for the great role they have played in helping the human race start to get its health back on the right track!

Contents

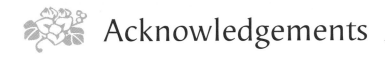

Acknowledgements

We would like to express our gratitude to the pioneers of the healthy approach to eating at the Bristol Cancer Help Centre. Above all, we would like to acknowledge the vision, dedication and generosity of those who created the centre — Penny and David Brohn and Pat and Christopher Pilkington. We honour the key roles played by the first medical director of the centre, Dr Alec Forbes, and the original nutritional therapist, Ute Brookman (who remains at the Centre to this day), in creating the dietary guidelines which have helped many thousands of people both fight and prevent cancer.

We would also like to acknowledge our lovely editors, Wanda Whiteley, Sam Grant and Claire Dunn for their faith in this project, and the production team at Thorsons for their great work in bringing this book into print.

DR ROSY DANIEL AND JANE SEN

Dr Rosy Daniel would also like to thank Jane Sen, her co-author, for being prepared to leave, temporarily, the glittering world of the celebrity chef to come to the Bristol Cancer Help Centre and revolutionize the food. She has used her tremendous skill and creativity to make vegan food both glamorous and accessible, and you will experience her brilliance for yourself as you explore her recipes in this book.

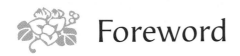

Foreword

We are what we eat. How many times have we all heard that simple health-education message and ignored its impact? Through aeons of evolutionary time, we as a race have survived and developed. But over the last 50 years, two sudden and major changes have taken place. We can now live much longer thanks to medical science, and this trend continues. But increasing affluence and new food technology – production, storage and preparation – has led to the average Western diet becoming distinctly unhealthy. This combination of increased life expectancy and a poor diet is leading to an unprecedented epidemic of potentially lethal diseases such as cancer, heart attacks and strokes. It has been estimated that 35 per cent of cancers are caused by an unhealthy diet, as are about 50 per cent of arterial disease cases. So what can we do about it? We need two things: motivation and information. This is where this very timely book by Rosy Daniel and Jane Sen comes in.

Here you will find some very practical advice. We in Britain are overfed with the wrong sorts of food – produced by an industry that spends millions of pounds each year on slick advertising and marketing strategies. A healthy diet need not be expensive. This easy-to-read guide tells you how to change your diet for the better.

The first chapter tells you why you should change your diet. Reducing total calorie intake to avoid obesity is an obsession with many, but it's *what* we eat as well as how much that is important. Dieting and bingeing are often written about, but are irrelevant to the long-term change in diet required to be healthy. The second chapter tells you how to make the necessary changes to your diet; the third chapter details what to change.

There is still much uncertainty about our food and its relationship to health. A small amount of alcohol may, for example, be beneficial. Eating lean meat may also be useful and is an excellent source of protein. But four principles, stressed time and again in this book, come over strongly in all serious studies of the subject:

1 reduce your intake of animal fat;
2 increase your daily fibre content;
3 eat plenty of fresh fruit and vegetables;
4 avoid obesity.

The fourth chapter deals with the concept of food as therapy. There is no doubt that conventional medicine has fastidiously avoided this area. Evidence of objective benefit is difficult to evaluate. But if a patient can feel better by changing his or her diet, then by definition this change has a positive effect. Increasingly, people with a wide range of illnesses want to experiment with their diet – it is part of the empowering process that puts the patient in the driving seat. This book provides some very safe and sound advice for us all.

KAROL SIKORA PHD, FRCR, FRCP, VISITING PROFESSOR OF CANCER MEDICINE, DEPT OF CANCER MEDICINE, IMPERIAL COLLEGE SCHOOL OF MEDICINE, HAMMERSMITH, LONDON.

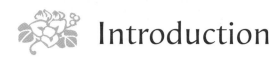

Introduction

Since its opening in 1980, the Bristol Cancer Help Centre has used healthy diet as a cornerstone of its approach to helping people with cancer recover their health. Former centre medical director, Dr Rosy Daniel, now feels adamant that this is the sort of diet all of us in the West should be adopting as a matter of urgency, to prevent cancer from starting in the first place. We know that cancer, arterial disease and probably rheumatoid arthritis, asthma and diabetes all have extremely strong dietary links, and that the main culprit is our excessive consumption of animal foods and sugary and processed foods and the relative lack of fruit, vegetables and non-processed whole foods. The problem is that although most of us know this, we are often very resistant to making the change to a healthy diet.

This resistance may be put down to a number of factors. Obviously there is the pleasure we all take in consuming rich, sweet foods. There can be great comfort in the instant gratification we can get from sweets, chocolates and takeaway foods. There is also the social pressure, at school, at work and in the home, to eat 'normal' foods so that we are not seen as fussy or difficult. In particular, there's pressure on parents to be good home-makers and to produce meals that win the immediate approval and affection of loved ones – sometimes at the cost of producing foods that are more healthy. And, of course, there is the negative image surrounding healthy food. How often have we heard it described as 'rabbit food' or 'hippy food', or becoming vegetarian equated with total deprivation!

This means that two things need to happen if we are to make the change successfully to a diet that's kinder to our bodies. The first is to help people change their diet in such a way that the change can be lasting, and does not result in stress or feeling as though they are missing out on 'nicer' foods. The second is linked to this – and is to change the image of healthy eating altogether!

The first of these objectives is our reason for writing this book, which I hope will serve as an extremely practical guide to the anti-cancer diet. The second of these objectives is tackled by our inspired chef, Jane Sen. Her delicious recipes are so good that healthy eating is guaranteed to become a pleasure.

We hope that, armed with this book, you will have the knowledge, guidance, support and inspiration to embark upon a new way of cooking and eating. This change will not only bring you good health but will also be a wonderful expression of your creativity and a great source of pleasure.

CHAPTER 1

Why Change the Way You Eat?

The Effects of Our Western Diet

It is now time for all of us who eat a typical Western diet to make the move to change the way we eat. Cancer and arterial disease (which causes heart attacks and strokes) are most strongly associated with our unhealthy eating patterns; people from Japan, China and Africa who take up a Western lifestyle and diet quickly start to demonstrate the same vulnerability to these lethal illnesses, having previously been protected by their more balanced diet.

Cancer and arterial disease now kill 75 per cent of British people.[1]

OUR DIET IS BADLY OUT OF PROPORTION

An unhealthy diet causes 35 per cent of cancer in the Western world, even more than can be attributed to smoking, which causes 30 per cent of cancer.[2] The problem is that our diet has evolved faster than our bodies' ability to cope with it. As we have grown more affluent, our diet has become richer in both fats and proteins, and has become more highly flavoured with salt, sugar, spices and additives. Simultaneously, food has become far more processed and refined, its valuable roughage and nutrients being taken out. We have also tended to eat fewer and fewer vegetables, cereals, pulses and fruits. This has created the bizarre, paradoxical situation in which we are both overfed *and* undernourished. The result is a chronic deterioration in our energy levels and in the body's immune system and ability to repair itself, which leads to a generalized increase in our susceptibility to disease.

In China, fat consumption makes up 13 per cent of the diet, as compared with 40 per cent in the UK; animal proteins account for only 7 per cent of all protein eaten as compared with 70 per cent in the UK, and coronary heart disease is lower by a ratio of 4:100 in China than the UK (that is, for every four heart-disease sufferers in China, there are 100 in the UK).[3]

Vegetarians are 40 per cent less likely to die from cancer[4] and 30 per cent less likely to die from cardiovascular disease.[5]

EXCESS FOOD AND ENERGY DEPLETION

The chronic excess of fat, protein, salt and sugar puts the body into a state of physiological stress and toxicity. This happens because our systems are designed in such a way that we can tolerate only a very small variation in the levels of these substances within our blood, otherwise the functioning of many of our delicate tissues, particularly the brain, goes haywire. In order to regulate the blood levels of these substances, the liver, kidney and pancreas have to work extremely hard. Not only do these processes cost the body a great deal of energy, but they also use up valuable minerals, vitamins and enzymes, depleting the body stores of these vital substances as a result. This exaggerates the depletion we already suffer as a result of our nutritionally impoverished diets.

In the short term, the effects of this process can be recognized by the drowsiness and nausea we may feel following a rich meal, which may inhibit our ability to function properly for an hour or two afterwards. But more sinister than this is the effect on our energy over the long term. The most common complaint faced by GPs nowadays is the new TATT syndrome: 'Tired All The Time'! Of course, we get into a vicious cycle here because the lethargy created by bad eating habits disinclines us to exercise properly, and this, coupled with sedentary jobs, stress and other bad habits such as drinking and smoking, precipitates us into a state of chronic exhaustion.

BODY BREAKDOWN

The problem does not stop here! Despite its best efforts, the body rarely can completely metabolize and excrete away the excess fat, protein, sugar and salt, so often its only recourse is to store these substances inappropriately in the cells or in deposits along the lining of the blood vessels themselves. This in turn leads to hardening of the arteries, fluid retention due to the ensuing imbalance of sodium, potassium and glucose in the cells, and even the depositing of proteins within the tissues (which may well contribute to antibody production and auto-immune processes, where the body starts to make antibodies against itself as occurs in such diseases as rheumatoid arthritis).

In these conditions, no tissues of the body can work well, and functioning at all levels becomes compromised; we also become fat and prone to cellulite, varicose veins, skin problems and long-term stress on our musculo-skeletal system. The skin itself is an organ of excretion, and many of the greasy skin problems and ensuing spots we suffer from in the West (for which we are sold billions of pounds' worth of cosmetics each year) arise from the skin playing its part in excreting excess fats and toxins. The effect of excess on the musculo-skeletal system is obviously seen in increased wear and tear on the system and the degenerative disease of osteoarthritis. The general stiffness many of us experience without actually having joint disease is also due to these deposits of excess fat, protein, sugar and salt.

GUT DISORDERS

Further to this, we have more problems created by the fact that we do not eat enough fibre, fruit, vegetables, cereals or pulses. The primary effect of this deficiency is on our bowel. The passage of food through the body is slowed down, which often leads to discomfort, abdominal distension, constipation and piles, and sometimes irritable bowel syndrome and diverticulitis. The secondary effect is that the slow transit time of food through the gut leaves far longer for any toxins present within food to be absorbed. It has been found that those on high-fibre diets who accidentally take in toxins or bacteria often stay well, while those on low-fibre diets get stomach upsets.

FOOD ABSORPTION

It takes several hours to digest the cellulose-bound nutrients in fruits, cereals, pulses and vegetables, meaning that after this type of meal there is a gentle trickle of nutrients into the body over a period of many hours. When a concentrated sugary or fatty food is eaten in an easily digestible form, such as glucose in a chocolate bar or fat coating a fried meal, this moves quickly into the bloodstream, causing an enormous peak in the levels of sugar and fat in the blood. The liver and pancreas work hard to reduce this peak quickly, resulting in the rapid change from a peak to a trough in the blood levels of these substances. This often creates irritability and more hunger, and a tendency to rush to other foods that may give quick gratification but again set off the vicious cycle described here.

MUCUS PRODUCTION

There is another marked effect of eating excess fat and protein, particularly as a result of a large intake of dairy foods: the production of a great deal of excess mucus – yet another way the body attempts to excrete the excess. This in turn leads to a tendency to infection, rheumatic illnesses and exacerbation of allergies. It might interest you to know that the Chinese word for cheese is 'solid mucus' – needless to say, milk products form a very small part of the traditional Chinese diet!

VITAMIN AND MINERAL DEFICIENCY

Of course, the other big problem about our low intake of fruits, vegetables, cereals and pulses is that these foods form the major source of vitamins and, particularly, minerals. These plant foods also have high levels of *essential fatty acids*, which are far better for us than the type of fatty acids found in meat. They are also rich in plant enzymes, which have a highly beneficial effect on our metabolic, growth and repair processes. The definition of the word 'vitamin' is 'vital for life' – need I say more?

Another phenomenon that occurs in the West is that our appetites can be subdued by foods which have plenty of calories but no nutritional value. For example, a chocolate bar may completely satisfy us but it has virtually nothing other than sugar in it. To get the same number of calories we would have to eat around 2.5 kilos (5 ½ lb) of apples; in the process we would also have given ourselves a huge amount of valuable vitamins, minerals, fibre and enzymes. This brings us back to the idea of being overfed and undernourished simultaneously.

All of the vitamins, minerals and essential fatty acids required by our bodies are vital for the correct functioning of our tissues. It is now clear that vitamins A, C and E (sometimes known as the antioxidant vitamins), in combination with the minerals zinc and selenium, play an especially important role in protecting us against cancer by deactivating dangerous *free radicals* – chemicals taken into and formed in the body as a result of pollution and dietary impurities. Free radicals attack lipids, proteins, enzymes and DNA, causing a variety of pathological problems and cancer. Vitamins are vital to protect the cells and to keep the cancer-producing 'free radical' chemicals produced by chemical carcinogens, radiation and the metabolic stress of an unhealthy diet from causing *oxidative damage* and transforming into cancer cells.

The recommended daily allowances of these substances as quoted by the medical profession are the amounts required to keep us free from deficiency diseases such as scurvy and rickets – we need far more to maintain positive health. A large proportion of our diet should be made up of fruit and vegetables, especially as petrochemical and other environmental pollution worsens. Many people now take antioxidants (in the form of vitamin/mineral supplements) regularly as a preventive; details of using vitamins and minerals in prevention and treatment are given in Chapter 4 of this book.

It seems that we have a great myth to break – that the more we eat, especially in terms of all those things that were once thought to be especially good for us, like milk, cheese, butter, cream and meat – the healthier we will be. In fact it is clear that the reverse is true, and that it is essential that we return to a diet far closer in nature to that of the poorer countries of the world, based predominantly on carbohydrates, pulses, nuts, vegetables and fruits, with a far lower intake of protein, sugar, fat and food additives.

The Quality of Food in 'Civilized' Society

Unfortunately, the disproportion of our Western diet is not the only problem. There is also the huge issue of how our food is produced, processed, packaged and stored, and hence what sort of shape it is in by the time it reaches our kitchens.

INTENSIVE FARMING

Most farmers have been forced through economic pressures into extremely intensive farming processes where high yield is achieved with chemicals, fertilizers and hormones which speed growth and add bulk.

Agriculture

Because of the pressure to produce crop after crop of vegetables out of the same land, there is a breakdown in the health and homeostasis of the soil, meaning that yet more chemicals are used to control diseases, pests and weeds. On a lettuce farm where I once worked through a summer holiday, the same piece of earth was used eight times each summer, new plants being planted within hours of the old ones being cut. For each crop the soil was sprayed six times – twice with weedkillers, twice with pesticides and twice with fertilizers. The more toxic pesticides were sprayed onto the bare soil, directly adjacent to young plants which were already growing and could not possibly have avoided contamination. This chemical onslaught occurs before the second round of sprays, gases and radiation used to keep fruit and vegetables perfect in transit!

The overall effect of these practices is that often growth is too quick for the usual nutrients to develop and become incorporated into the plants; this problem is exacerbated because the soil is already low in vital trace elements because of repeated usage. So the vegetables may look perfect but be tasteless, watery or even hollow inside in the case of some carrots; certainly they do not contain the nutrients we would expect to find in them. To boot, these vegetables have been found to contain the chemicals used to stimulate their growth and protect them from bugs. It is impossible to wash these substances off and avoid contaminating ourselves with toxic chemicals (although careful washing will help remove the surface chemicals used once the product has grown).

Banning of organochlorine pesticide Lindane in Israel has brought the overall incidence of breast cancer down by 8 per cent, and the rate in the lowest age group down by 24 per cent.[6]

Animal Husbandry

In animals, growth-stimulating factors such as steroids and hormones may be used (often illegally) to speed growth, add muscle bulk and increase milk and egg production. Drugs are also used to control pests and disease. As with humans, these practices weaken the ability of the animal to eradicate disease and infection. These substances may be found in high quantities within the meat, and particularly the liver, of the animal, and of course may be passed at higher levels, dissolved in fat or through the animal's milk into dairy foods as the animal itself excretes the chemicals. (These substances become most concentrated in high-fat foods such as cheese and cream.) Added to this is the effect of contaminating pesticides and fertilizers on the grass the animals eat and in the feed and water they are given, which will also pass to humans through animal products – particularly those products high in fat.

There is another issue here, too: the potential for transmission of infection from animal food. Being far closer in our make-up to animals than to the plant kingdom, we are likely to be prone to similar infecting agents. Animal foods put us at risk of infection from bacteria such as salmonella (eggs), listeria (cheese), and viruses such as BSE from beef. These are the ones we know about – I feel sure many other mystery diseases of our time will be found to have their origins in infections transmitted in this way.

The recent human and economic disasters created first by BSE and then by foot and mouth disease have shown us just how much modern farming and slaughter techniques leave the food chain open to infection. It is my belief that a great deal more cancer comes through the viral infection of food than we currently realize. We already know that 15 per cent of cancers result from viral infection – most frequently, cancers of the cervix, liver primaries and many of the lymphomas and leukaemias can be caused in this way. My hunch is that within the next decade, links will be found connecting many other common cancers to viruses and other infectious agents as the association between cancer and the animal food chain is so high.

We see, therefore, that modern food production leaves us with food of a lower nutritional value, which may also be quite polluted, toxic, infectious and antigenic. Many members of the older generation complain about the tastelessness of much of our vegetables, fruits and meats, and the way that bulk-produced chicken even tastes of fish (as it is often fed on fish meal). Indeed, anyone who has ever grown their own vegetables will be staggered by the difference between the taste of fresh, home-grown vegetables and the beautiful but nutritionally pale imitations which are generally on offer in our shops.

FOOD PROCESSING

Sadly, the processing of food, which occurs to transform the raw material into highly marketable goodies of one sort or another, further damages it by removing much of the fibre, roughage and essential nutrients. Much processing came about through the fashion for 'refining' food – turning brown flour white, brown rice white and brown sugar white. In the process many important vitamins, minerals and *co-factors* (required to promote the activity of other substances, such as vitamins) are lost. In addition to this, there is the further destruction of vitamins and enzymes during the heating and sterilizing processes; the addition of chemicals in the processes of bleaching, dyeing, flavouring, emulsifying and stabilizing; not to mention the effects of plastic containers and *gamma-irradiation*. Plastic containers and bottles are believed to release potentially toxic chemicals into their contents, and nowadays many foods, especially fruits, vegetables and spices, are irradiated to prevent decay. Little is known as yet about the potential dangers and nutritional loss of this practice.

However, what becomes clear when we look at the frighteningly long sell-by dates on many packaged and processed foods, is that the foods have been rendered virtually inert nowadays. It is very much in the producers' interests to control all the normal decaying processes, but the risk is that the life is knocked completely out of the food and we are left with a chemical corpse rather than a living, vibrant, natural food. The most vivid illustration of this can be seen using Kirlian photography, which shows us visually the vital energy radiating from matter. An organic brown loaf has an energy field several centimetres deep, whereas a white processed loaf has no energy field at all!

We may go on to add insult to injury in the types of cooking methods we use. For example, frying foods at very high temperatures tends to de-nature them, as most enzymes and vitamins cannot withstand high temperatures. In the process, dangerous and unstable free radicals are produced in the fat and in the food being cooked. Even worse is barbecuing, when the presence of *hydrocarbons* in the smoke accelerates this process, especially in the cooking of meat. The curing of meat with *salt petre* (as in many salamis) is also dangerous because the sodium nitrite can change to carcinogenic nitrosamines in the gut.

Microwaving food may have similarly destructive effects, as microwaves are extremely high energy and heat the food to higher temperatures than most frying techniques. This is why microwaved foods must always be left to stand, as otherwise the high energy will be dissipated in our gullet and stomach with potentially dangerous consequences. Freezing food is not intrinsically bad, although food does deteriorate in the freezer over time and the freezer should not be used to store food for months on end.

The net result of modern-day food production, therefore, is that it provides us with food which may look wonderful but which may be more dead than alive, lacking in nutrients, contaminated with chemicals and growth factors, and with a very low fibre content to boot.

WATER

It is also likely that the water we drink from our taps may be seriously contaminated. Many water authorities do not yet routinely measure for by-products of the plastics, petrochemical and farming industries. Organochlorines, for example, may mimic hormones and could possibly be responsible for the dramatic rise in hormone-related cancers (most commonly lung, breast and prostate). Of course, foods and water may be pronounced safe, but this is only valid when the presence of contaminants is known about and measured, when the effects of these contaminants are known, and of course when those with a commercial interest do not suppress the distribution of information!

The Quantity of Food We Eat

Most of us in the West simply eat far too much. Over 60 per cent of British adults are overweight, and the proportion is even higher in the US. In fact, it has been said that the amount spent on slimming products in the richer countries of the world could easily solve the problem of starvation in Third World countries. Our hunger can be satisfied with relatively modest amounts of food, but we go on and on eating for all sorts of other reasons. This would not be so bad if the foods we were eating were high in fibre and low in calories, but usually the reverse is true. The obesity created is obviously a problem. It makes us less mobile and far less inclined to exercise. This in turn renders us more sluggish, with accompanying deterioration of our posture. Joints suffer and the tendency to arthritic problems is aggravated. We are also put at risk of high blood pressure and poor circulation, and become an anaesthetic risk if we require surgery.

We are also afflicted by the damage to our self-image that being fat creates, and carry the further burdens of stress, dieting and bingeing. On top of all these well-known problems of obesity is the newer association being made between obesity and cancer risk. Originally, it was noted anecdotally that women in P.O.W. camps on poor diets had almost no breast cancer. The relationship between high calorie intake and cancer of the breast, prostate, colon and ovary has since been demonstrated. Animal studies have shown that a reduction in food intake by 30 per cent stopped all tumour growth and doubled the life expectancy of the animals. Further animal studies have shown that decreasing the amounts of protein, sugar and fat in the diet reduces tumour growth directly and exponentially.

While it has been almost impossible to repeat these studies on humans (as it is hard to expect a randomized group to remain on a low-calorie diet for long periods of time in order to measure the possible effect on tumour development), it has certainly become clear that fat is strongly associated with many cancers, particularly the hormonal cancers (breast, ovary, uterus, prostate, testicular), and also colon cancer. The association is far stronger with animal fats than vegetable fats, and the overall incidence of cancer is much higher in the rich countries than the poor ones. Fat is seen not as initiating cancer, but as promoting it once it exists in the body.

The American Cancer Society say that the overweight have a 50 per cent
higher incidence of cancer.

It is known that fatty tissue produces hormones, and it may well be through this mechanism alone that being overweight creates extra cancer risk. Alternatively, as mentioned before, it may be due to chemical pollutants present in the animal fats we are taking in either directly in meat or through dairy produce. Animal fat contains both the animal's own hormones and other growth-stimulating substances used to promote its growth and milk production, or chemicals ingested from feeds, grass or water. In short, both the animal's fat and our own fat become manufacturers and stores of potentially harmful substances which are putting us at higher risk of cancer. It is worth pointing out here that the fat in chicken and fish, unlike that in other meats, is stored more exclusively under their skin than in their flesh, so it is easier to eliminate before cooking (by removing and discarding the skin) if desired.

DRINKS

Sweetened drinks and alcohol are a major source of extra calories and obesity in the West. Twenty years ago, most people drank water with their meals, and alcohol or sweetened drinks were reserved for special occasions. Nowadays it is not uncommon for individuals to take in an extra 1,000 calories a day through fizzy 'pop', beer, wine and spirits, mixers and the milk and sugar in tea and coffee. Again we are in the trap of 'empty calories' – becoming satisfied by substances with almost no nutritional value, making ourselves fat in the process.

How We Eat

Next we must face the question of how we eat and therefore how able we are to digest our food and gain nutritional benefit from it. In order to digest and absorb food properly, we must be relaxed. When we are stressed, rushed or preoccupied with other things, our nervous system is in a state of arousal. This favours the operation of our brain and muscles – in other words the organs of doing and thinking, fight and flight. This happens at the expense of the internal housekeeping functions of the body, which cannot work optimally unless we are in a relaxed state and the 'attention' of our organism can be directed into digestion, absorption, metabolism, immune function, growth and repair. This means that we can be eating quite good food but only be getting a small proportion of its nutritional benefits. An extreme example of this is seen in the failure-to-thrive syndrome in babies, where their growth is inhibited by the fear and anxiety they suffer as a result of lack of physical contact, bonding and love. In this state, absorption of food and actual growth come to a virtual standstill.

In our stressed, rushed modern lifestyles, when many meals are eaten on the hoof, in the car, while talking on the telephone and doing 20 other things, our digestion and nutrition are severely compromised. Whether we stop to eat and enjoy our food or not can become one of the clearest signs of whether we are literally able to give ourselves space and time to nourish ourselves at the physical level, let alone emotionally and spiritually.

COMFORT EATING

Food is very commonly used as an emotional prop, both for comfort and to take away difficult feelings – by eating or not eating. For some, a sense of control in life is re-established through the withholding of food, sometimes to the point of anorexia. Rich, sweet and fatty foods have a sedative effect on us because of their toxicity and the work the body has to do to restore equilibrium. Food for some may therefore be taking the place of tranquillizers! Many people discover when they try to change their diet, omitting the unhealthier foods, that they are suddenly faced with emotions and feelings they have been suppressing for years, with which they feel unable to cope.

This sort of situation can lead to addictive dependency on food in just the same sort of way that people become dependent on drink or drugs. It can even sometimes be seen that people become addicted to foods to which they are actually quite allergic, because the symptoms and drowsiness they experience while their body is dealing with the challenge relieve them temporarily of some of their anxiety or other painful feelings. This can be exploited by others, who can control them through 'comfort feeding'. Many people keep their families dependent on and attached to them, trading unconsciously on the power of control that overfeeding gives them.

SOCIAL EATING

Another distorting factor in the relationship between what we eat and what our bodies need is the extensive use of food in social situations. Most entertaining revolves almost exclusively around food and drink, and often party food is almost entirely made up of pastries, cakes, crisps, biscuits and fried and barbecued foods, all washed down with large amounts of very sweet fizzy drinks and alcohol. In these types of situations we may be taking in our calorific requirement for a whole day in one sitting!

Eating in restaurants is the most common leisure-time activity, and of course fast food is always available on the street, at home, or delivered to your door at all hours of the day and night . To make things worse, often the insecure host or hostess will aim to please, and go on feeding guests more and more, using food as an entertainment or as a way of augmenting a lack of social skills! By far the majority of food eaten in social contexts has nothing at all to do with our nutritional needs, and forms a great part of the distorting influence on our health and lifestyle.

EATING PATTERNS THROUGH THE DAY

As well as the problem of eating our food quickly while we are preoccupied, there is a growing tendency to leave the largest meal until very late in the day. Often breakfast is reduced to a cup of coffee, and lunch a quick sandwich; dinner becomes the serious meal of the day. This plays havoc with the metabolism of the body, because during the part of the day when we have the biggest need for energy, it is having to be produced from stored substances such as glycogen and fat. Whereas at night, when we are sleeping, the body is being flooded with available energy sources from the large meal we have just eaten. The problem with this appears to be that not only is the work of storing and liberating the energy-producing nutrients being done twice, but that we end up storing more than we use. This is because at times of very low blood sugar during the day, the body moves into very efficient 'fasting' metabolic mode, liberating as little of the stored nutrients as it can. The net result is that we gain weight, as more and more food will be laid down during the night as fat, and less will be changed back during the day to glucose for available energy supply.

It is therefore very important that we revert to either the more continental habit of eating the main meal at midday, with only a snack during the evening; or even to the traditional Eastern habit of having the largest meal at breakfast time. Again, the prime requirement here is that we slow down and make eating an important part of our day.

DIETING AND BINGEING – FIGHTING FASHION

One of the greatest jokes of our time is that despite the fact that 60 per cent of society is overweight, fashion continues to portray the image of lean, firm-fleshed, healthy-looking slim people as the ideal towards which we must all strive. In fact, many models are so thin that they are clearly bordering on anorexia. This would seem to point to the underlying revulsion we feel with our out-of-control bodies and eating habits. The media clearly taps into and exploits this self-hatred, perpetually encouraging us to invest in clothes, beauty products and slimming aids to attain this state of 'perfection'.

All studies of the effects of dieting have shown that the most common outcome of dieting is a phase of bingeing with a rapid return to the original weight, or an even higher weight than when the diet was started. This may well be in part due to the problem described earlier – that when we eat less our body goes into 'fasting mode' and can become very efficient at eking out its supplies. This means that as soon as we start eating more again the extra is deposited as fat.

Glamorous comedienne Dawn French has worked hard to try to encourage larger women to feel comfortable and attractive just the way they are by continually pointing out the fact that 47 per cent of women in Britain are a size 16 or over! While it is laudable to help women feel better about themselves and to break the crazy cycle of dieting and bingeing that most women in the West permanently find themselves in, it is inescapable that obesity is linked with disease of all kinds. A healthy way of returning to a good weight is to combine better eating habits with the necessary emotional support and proper exercise.

The Environment

The other vital reason we must change the way we eat is the effect our eating habits are having on the environment. In the days when food was grown locally using low-energy technology, and eaten in the communities by whom it was grown, the average input of energy was 1 kilojoule per 8 kilojoules of food energy being produced. Nowadays, because of the energy used in intensive farming – the running and making of machinery and fertilizers, transportation, processing, packaging and transportation of food to the shops (possibly right across the world), handling of the goods within shops, and transportation of the public to and from the shops to buy the food – there is now an input of 50 kilojoules of energy in food production for every kilojoule of food energy produced![7] This is an extremely dramatic statistic and makes it abundantly clear that we are on a destructive course towards the exhaustion of available energy resources.

However, most of what distorts this picture so greatly is the big shift towards the consumption of animal foods, which require so much more energy to produce than plant foods. For example, it requires 10 times the energy input per pound of beef to produce the equivalent nutritional quantity of grain. In other words, we could feed 10 times as many people on a vegetarian diet than on a meat diet! The message is equally clear from the environment: we have to revert to eating a diet based upon vegetable rather than animal foods, which is grown organically and produced locally. Of course, the most local place of all is our own garden, and this is the ideal solution – to start growing our own vegetables organically at home if we have any land whatsoever.

Cancer, Diet and the Immune and Repair Systems

The important question for those with cancer and those wishing to prevent cancer is 'how does an unhealthy diet relate to getting cancer, and how can changing my diet prevent cancer or stabilize cancer once it occurs?'

The specific links with diet and cancer concern eating meat and animal fats, and too few vitamins, minerals and plant foods (which contain vital plant chemicals known as *phytochemicals*). A vegetarian diet provides greater protection from cancer due to higher levels of fibre, decreased fat, or increased consumption of a wide range of the phytochemicals present in plant foods.

- Vegetarians are 40 per cent less likely to die from cancer.[4]
- The incidence of breast cancer is 30 per cent lower in those who do not consume animal fat.[1]
- The incidence of colon cancer is 25 per cent lower in those who do not consume animal fat.[1]

The non-specific factors include low energy levels, depletion in the body of important vitamins, minerals and essential fatty acids due to poor diet, and the poor functioning of tissues as a result of this and chronic toxicity. This, of course, is exacerbated by stress and the resulting poor absorption of food. As mentioned before, those who study disease in populations assess that 35 per cent of all cancer is caused by the Western diet; another 30 per cent by smoking.[2] This means that 65 per cent of all cancer could be eradicated if we started taking a more responsible attitude towards our own health.

Broadly speaking, it would appear that it is substances in meat and fats that promote cancer, and the action of vitamins and minerals which protect us against these and other pollutants in our environment. A high-fibre diet helps by limiting absorption of cancer-producing factors. The active enzymes in raw plant foods also convey protection and health. Vitamins and minerals have direct stimulant effects on our immune system, and it is postulated that vitamins and minerals can stabilize and inhibit the growth of tumour cells directly.

All the repair and healing systems of the body are dependent upon good nutrition and a balanced diet, as everything from control of bleeding and the healing of wounds to the fighting of infection depends upon the correct balance of vitamins, minerals, adequate energy and protein back-up to take place effectively. In an overloaded toxic system, normal tissue function will be impaired – the function of the immune and repair systems included.

Another significant factor is that the body will attend first to stress or emergency situations. The excess of fat, salt, sugar or protein in the body constitutes a physiological emergency, and while this situation persists, immune and repair functions will be compromised as the resources of the body go towards achieving homeostasis at the expense of immune function. A smaller but important factor is that when there is a great deal of extremely diverse material being fed into the body, particularly of tissue which is close in structure to our own, a great part of the immune system's function will be diverted towards recognizing these foreign tissues and making antibodies against them. Again, it is theorized that this may be a cause of some of the mystery illnesses of our time, as the antigenic stimulus from animal tissue may lead to the formation of antibodies to our own tissues, as occurs in the case of auto-immune diseases such as rheumatoid arthritis, thyroid disease and diabetes. Overactivity in terms of auto-antibody production and surveillance of 'invading proteins' from outside may distract the immune function from adequate surveillance of 'the enemy within' – that is, the formation of cancer cells – or create inflammation of tissues, creating an ideal environment for the development of cancer.

However, it has already been mentioned that in a stressed, frightened, preoccupied individual, the functioning of the immune and repair systems becomes secondary to responding to a threat in our environment, as a result of which most of us in the West have our immune function compromised already.

In the US there have been government guidelines since 1983 suggesting that to prevent cancer it is essential that we cut down our fat intake and increase our consumption of vegetables, fruit and fibre, and decrease our consumption of alcohol, food additives and smoked foods. In Britain, due to the pressure of the agriculture and food industries, and resistance from the medical profession, these guidelines have only been issued since 1998, and then in a very low-key fashion.

A database of scientific research on diet and cancer compiled by the Bristol Cancer Help Centre[8] during the mid-1990s contains around 6,000 peer-reviewed studies performed over the preceding 14-year period, and clearly points to the connection between the way we eat and our tendency to cancer. This database is available for study by those with an academic interest in this subject. The relationship between food, the way we eat and cancer could not be clearer from this mass of evidence, and for me the question 'Why change the way we eat?' has been answered definitively. To diminish the risk of cancer and all other diseases of civilization, and the abuse that our over-indulgent diet causes to our environment, we must all now rethink the way we eat as a matter of urgency.

Let us move on, then, to the question of how we go about it.

CHAPTER 2

How to Change the Way You Eat

Some people, given the information about the need to change their way of eating, go away and achieve this in one fell swoop. I have known people who have learned about the role of diet in preventing cancer and have gone round their kitchen with a black bin bag, emptied into it half the contents of their fridges, freezers and cupboards and started their new way of eating the very same day! I would have to say that this is a small minority, because for most of us changing the way we eat is very difficult due to lack of information about what to buy and how to go about preparing it. There are also time and money considerations, and emotional investment in our food and the way we eat (not to mention sabotage, however well meant, from our families and friends).

The most important thing is that the change is lasting and that you will not set yourself up for failure and stress, which would, of course, be entirely counter-productive to your overall state of wellbeing. It is therefore helpful if you are as well prepared as you can be before making the change, by anticipating your need for support, sufficient information, clarity and resolution about the exact approach you are going to follow, and specific advice about your own personal needs if you have medical problems affecting your eating, digestion, weight or excretion.

Preparation

The first key to achieving anything is having sufficient support to do it! Usually the best place to start is by discussing your dietary changes with those close to you, particularly those you live with or regularly share meals with. The ideal scenario is that your friends and family might change with you, as clearly this is an issue for everybody. If they cannot agree to join you, get them to agree at least not to sabotage you by offering you things which will make it difficult or, if you are the main cook, by expecting you to cook two different meals. The availability of many vegetarian food substitutes which imitate meat products (such as veggie burgers, soya sausages, mince and stewing steak) make it very much easier to take a reluctant family along with you.

Once you have got your new way of eating established, be prepared to ask friends over and show them how you eat by cooking for them. It may also encourage them to take these steps themselves! Be prepared to take healthy food with you to work, and again sit back and watch how others begin to catch on to the idea.

You may decide to take a course in whole-food cookery. Many adult education centres offer reasonably priced lessons where you can learn more about cooking with delicious health-giving ingredients.

You may also have recognized, in the section on 'Comfort Eating' in Chapter 1, that changing the way you eat is going to bring up a lot of difficult feelings or make you feel very insecure. If this should happen, it might be wise to see a counsellor. As your previously suppressed emotions arise, you will then have the opportunity of processing them and integrating them into the positive changes you are making for yourself. The benefits will then be doubled, as you will be tackling your physical and emotional state simultaneously. It is very important to take this seriously because, as with the dieting and bingeing cycle, unless the underlying emotions are sorted out, your efforts to change may well be thwarted.

Information

The second key to success is to have all the relevant information at your fingertips. Hopefully, by the time you have read this book, you will feel this is the case, but if not you may consider visiting a nutritional therapist to talk further so that your questions can be answered as you go along.

The information you will need is:

- clear dietary guidelines explaining what to eat and what not to eat
- a clear idea of what foods are available and what you should go out and buy
- an introductory meal plan to take you through the first few weeks
- nutritional information to ensure that what you are eating is balanced and healthy
- a good set of recipes.

All these areas will be explained in full in Chapter 3 together with meal plans, and recipes which can be found in Chapter 5.

The third key to success is to be very clear about your goals. By this I mean that once you have taken on board the information about the anti-cancer diet, you need to decide for yourself how far you are going to go, over what sort of period of time, and in what order. You may also wish to start the process with a 'spring-cleaning' diet (see Chapter 4), a fast or a period on juices, or alternatively you may wish to move into the process very slowly, making one small change at a time. The entire process will be explained under the heading 'Planning' in Chapter 3.

If you already have cancer, the fourth important step is to talk to a holistic doctor or experienced nutritional therapist. If you have a cancer which is causing problems with eating, swallowing, digestion, absorption or excretion of food, or if you have weight problems, the doctor or therapist should guide you in modifying your dietary changes to ensure you are getting adequate food, maintaining or putting on weight, and coping with any digestive problems.

Another major consideration here is chemotherapy and radiotherapy to the bowel. Chemotherapy causes slowing down of the bowel's activity and irritation of the lining of the bowel, which will create the need for soothing, relatively low-fibre foods during the time you are receiving this treatment. Radiation involving the bowel may also inhibit its function temporarily, and again care may be needed to adjust to a lower-fibre diet. By and large, nearly everyone changing to a healthier diet says that their bowel function improves within a few weeks, including those with a colostomy! However, it is wise if you have this or other problems to talk to the doctor first.

Making the Change Easier

Ideally, changing the way you eat should be treated as a process of exploration and creativity – an adventure rather than a process of deprivation! The world of vegetables, fruits, cereals and pulses is an extremely rich one. There are thousands and thousands of wonderful vegetarian dishes from all over the world to experiment with. Do not forget – the majority of the world's population lives on a largely vegetarian diet, and people such as Madhur Jaffrey have opened up the world of Eastern and Middle Eastern vegetarian food to us, as have many other authors describing Mexican, Italian, Spanish, Chinese, Indonesian and French vegetarian cooking.

The other thing I can promise categorically is that you will feel better once you start eating more healthily. Invariably, those who make this step say they are brighter, more energetic and happier, and wake up more easily – not to mention all the other sorts of positive improvements in health, such as possibly clearing up allergies such as hay fever, asthma and rheumatoid arthritis. The skin becomes clearer and usually excess fat gradually drops away. If you do already have cancer, it is better that you have medical supervision to make sure all is going as it should and that excess weight loss is being avoided.

One way to avoid feeling that you are in a process of deprivation is to start by *adding* things to your diet before you start to take things away. The obvious place to start is by increasing your intake of fruit, making sure that you have a minimum of two pieces of fruit a day. Next, be sure that you are eating vegetables twice a day, and/or salad with most of your meals. Experiment with different ways of cooking vegetables so they become more and more interesting, and also with different types of salads so that these can become a bigger part of your way of eating.

The next thing to do is to start changing one meal at a time to comply with the dietary guidelines. Most people start with breakfast, as this is the easiest meal to change over, and go on to lunch and then dinner. Again, learn new skills before cutting away your old way of eating, and get to the stage where you know enough vegetable recipes to fill a whole week before you make the complete changeover. Establish a master shopping list of the things you are likely to need each week. Then use this as a master checklist before you go shopping (there is an example of one in Chapter 3).

Some people find that if they have five established main meal recipes which are quick and easy for weekdays, they can then use the weekend to experiment with new recipes.

During this process it is hoped that a subtler change will start to take place in your ability to care and nurture yourself with food. The holistic healing process involves becoming better and better acquainted with yourself and your needs. Learning how to feed yourself sensitively and properly becomes an absolutely concrete symbol of this more loving relationship with yourself, which you will then be able to introduce into more and more areas of your life. This does not only apply to feeding ourselves with good-quality, well-balanced nutrition, but also with the colours and textures of our foods and the rich creative process involved in thinking about it, shopping for it, making it and serving it.

Bringing Attention to Food

Of course, there is the question of how we eat our food. As discussed earlier, it is clear that most of us need to set aside far more time for eating and digesting our food. I would strongly encourage you to return to the old rituals of setting the table and presenting food well, or creating your own rituals around food to enhance your enjoyment of it. Try not to rush away from the table as soon as possible – follow the example of our European neighbours who often take an hour after meals at the table relaxing and enjoying the company of family and friends. If you are alone, perhaps you could try and relax or read a book after eating rather than rushing off to do the next thing.

In these ways our food can begin to feed us on many levels – in terms of our creativity, our sensuality and our spirituality – and, like the Japanese tea ceremony, feeding ourselves can become a form of meditation. You will find that the more focus, attention and love you give to preparing your food, the more wonderful it will taste and the more deeply it will feed you and heal you.

I once found myself in a macrobiotic restaurant in Rotterdam, Holland, called Zonnemaire. With each course that arrived I became more amazed at the quality of the food, but this was not only quality in Egon Ronay terms, but in the attention and love that had gone into preparing the meal. Each course was exquisitely presented, culminating in a plate of fruit salad made as a miniature garden, with tiny branches of redcurrants standing as little trees among beautifully sculpted fruit and flowers. By the end of the meal I knew I was in the company of a very, very special chef. I asked to visit the kitchen and discovered that the chef was a Zen monk whose entire meditation was the growing, preparing and serving of food. He allowed no chatting in his kitchen, and all his staff (who adored him) worked in a gentle, focused, loving and highly creative spirit. As he sent each meal up in the lift to the restaurant he personally blessed the food, and it was obviously his love, blessing and the attention he gave to the whole process that communicated itself in every mouthful.

We hear also of the macrobiotic advice to chew each mouthful 50 times, giving full attention to the flavour and texture of the food while rendering it extremely digestible too. While this level of focus is not perhaps compatible with everyday living, we should aim to bring some of this quality of attention and consciousness into the way we prepare and eat our food, which will of course bring us into a far healthier relationship with ourselves, our food and our life process.

CHAPTER 3

What to Change in the Way You Eat

For health and cancer prevention, the ideal diet is whole-food, organic and vegan, supplemented with occasional organic fish, poultry and eggs. The underlying nutritional change we should be seeking to make is to increase the amount of vegetables, fruits, cereals, pulses (and therefore fibre) we take in, and to decrease our intake of protein, fat, salt, sugar, chemical additives and stimulants. This will result in a cleaner, lighter, less challenging diet which provides optimum levels of nutrients and energy in forms with which the body can cope most easily.

The results of changing to this diet will be a rapid increase in energy, greater mental clarity, an improvement in skin and bowel functioning, and reduction in symptoms such as nausea, heartburn, constipation and piles. Changing the diet in this way may also have pronounced benefits for those with existing medical problems such as arthritis, asthma, eczema and diabetes, sometimes resulting in complete remission of these conditions.

Another vital benefit of a healthy diet for those receiving medical treatment for cancer is that treatment becomes far easier to tolerate. The body can deal much more efficiently with the toxicity produced by chemotherapy and radiotherapy if there is a greatly reduced toxic load from the diet. Those who have had these treatments while first on an ordinary diet and then on a healthy diet have said that the level of nausea and debilitation they have suffered while being treated has diminished significantly. So, ideally, dietary changes should precede cancer treatment. How this translates into what we actually eat is as follows:

Recommended Foods

1 Whole foods: All food should be eaten whole, with nothing added or taken away –
   e.g. wholemeal bread, brown rice, brown flour.
2 Fresh fruit and vegetables (not tinned or frozen) should be eaten with every meal,
   especially green, leafy vegetables – e.g. cabbage, broccoli, sprouts. Aim to have a
   minimum of five servings of fruit and vegetables each day.
3 Raw food – vegetables, fruit and raw cereals, nuts and seeds. Try to eat some daily as
   salads, fruit salads, muesli or freshly prepared fruit juices – e.g. a mixture of carrot,
   apple and beetroot.
4 Organically grown food, as available and affordable.
5 High-fibre – e.g. beans, pulses, lentils, vegetables and cereals.
6 Cold-pressed oils for dressings and cooking.
7 Variety: Avoid depending on any one food excessively.

Foods to Increase Protein Intake if Required:

1 Fish and poultry (and game) – deep-sea fish is preferable, as is organically raised
   free-range poultry.
2 Eggs – organic free-range, maximum two per week.

Avoid as Much as Possible (especially if intensively farmed):

1 Red meat – beef, pork, lamb, veal, bacon, kidneys, liver, salamis and meat pâtés.
2 Dairy produce – cheese, butter, cream, yoghurt and milk (use soya products
   instead).

Avoid Excess:

3 Sugar
4 Salt
5 Fat – particularly animal fats such as butter, and meat fats.
6 Protein – 55g/2oz per day is adequate, unless you experience sudden weight loss.

7 Preservatives and additives, smoked or pickled foods – particularly barbecued foods.

8 Caffeine – tea, coffee, chocolate, cola, alcohol, nicotine and non-prescribed drugs.

9 Food which has been stored for long periods, irradiated, dried, processed, microwaved or repeatedly reheated.

Questions Answered

Some questions arise repeatedly regarding these guidelines. I have listed the most common ones here.

IS EATING BRAN A GOOD WAY TO INCREASE MY FIBRE INTAKE?

The answer to this is a categoric *No*. Pure bran is made up of fibre and almost nothing else and is highly irritant to the bowel. This is going from one extreme to the other; some studies have shown that bran is so irritant that it may actually be carcinogenic! It is quite sufficient to eat increased fibre as it occurs naturally in whole foods such as cereals, muesli, porridge, vegetables, pulses and whole-wheat flours and brown rice.

WHAT KIND OF FAT IS HEALTHY FOR THE BODY, AND IS MARGARINE REALLY BETTER THAN BUTTER?

The body does require fat in the diet – indeed there are substances called *essential fatty acids (see Glossary)* on which we are as dependent as vitamins for health. The best-known sources of these essential fatty acids are fish oil, evening primrose oil and linseed oil, but in fact they are found in many seeds and nuts. The fats to avoid are the saturated fats found in animal foods, which will be particularly concentrated in butter, cheese, cream, milk, yoghurt and of course meat fat (unless you buy very low-fat versions of these foods and are meticulous about cutting the fat off the meat you eat). Even so, these foods are also very high in protein and daily intake usually pushes us into protein excess. The animal fats have been specifically linked to both cancer and heart disease. The recommendation, therefore, is to move to unsaturated fats such as vegetable oils, particularly cold-pressed olive oil for cooking purposes, and even then to keep consumption within reasonable limits to avoid excess weight gain.

The problem with butter and margarine is that many commercially produced margarines are highly processed and contain *hydrogenated* and trans fatty acids, which are also unhealthy for the body. These are produced by the processing and excessive heating of the fats in the production process. Because of this problem many people have given up and reverted to butter. However, there are margarines – such as Vitaquel and Granose – which do not contain hydrogenated fatty acids. These should be the preferred choice, as they are a good source of unsaturated fatty acids.

Essential fatty acids are not only vital for health, but have also been seen to have a specific role in cancer prevention and treatment. There are two families of essential fatty acids – the omega-6 fatty acids and the omega-3 fatty acids. The omega-6s are found in high concentrations in evening primrose oil, and the omega-3s in particularly high concentrations in linseed oil, fish oils and game. It is the omega-3s which have the most protective effect, and for this reason those with cancer are well advised to add a dessertspoon of organic cold-pressed linseed oil to their food three times a day for its protective effect (not the type of linseed oil used for the cricket bat, however, as this contains petrol!).

At one time the advice was to take linseed oil with sulphur-containing proteins such as those found in cottage cheese. However, subsequent studies have shown that it is as effectively absorbed with other foods, and can be added to soups, dressings or rice. Another way to take linseed oil is by grinding linseed yourself in a clean coffee grinder: 2 dessertspoons of seed provide about the equivalent of 1 dessertspoon of the oil, and again this should be taken three times daily sprinkled over food.

WHEN MIGHT I NEED TO SUPPLEMENT MY DIET WITH MEAT, FISH OR EGGS, AND IF SO, WHAT SORT OF MEAT, FISH OR EGGS SHOULD I BUY?

Contrary to popular belief (verging on brainwashing by a combination of our mothers and the milk and meat marketing boards) it is perfectly possible for us to exist on a vegan diet without fading away or becoming ill! Remember – great big animals like elephants, cows, whales and apes all survive on purely plant diets, which may encourage you to have more faith in the vegan approach!

However, if you have cancer, your treatment may call for quite specific protein requirements – perhaps due to excessive weight loss or excessive tissue loss because of surgery or chemotherapy, or because the cancer involved is a type that produces a great deal of protein-containing fluid which has to be drained off, with consequent loss of protein from the body. In these instances it can become important to increase the protein intake with chicken, fish and eggs. It is always advisable to discuss this with a holistic doctor or nutritional therapist.

If your lifestyle involves intense physical activity, there is again likely to be an increased demand by the body for proteins to build muscle tissue. This would apply to athletes, gymnasts and those involved in hard physical work. But even here it should be noted that Olympic long-distance runners are now using a low-protein/high-carbohydrate diet after witnessing the great success of the Chinese runners who follow this type of diet (only eating fish twice weekly)! Again, professional advice may be sought in order to achieve the correct balance in your own situation.

When buying meat, fish or eggs, the emphasis must be on choosing organic. As already mentioned in Chapter 1, animals take in and concentrate in their tissues chemicals and growth-stimulating factors, and of course all animals raised with intensive farming techniques are likely to contain toxic chemical factors of one sort or another. When shopping, be clear about the distinction between free-range and organic. Although free-range eggs and meat may come from animals that have been free to run around, they may also have been fed pure chemical food! When buying fish, go for wild fish rather than farmed or processed fish, as farmed fish will have been given chemically augmented food and may have been processed with dyes and flavourings. For example, much smoked haddock and salmon is artificially coloured and flavoured. The best fish is therefore deep-sea fish and shellfish which have not been farmed. Deep-sea fish include sole, plaice, cod, haddock, red mullet, bass, turbot, John Dorey and hake, all of which can form an excellent source of very high-quality, easily digestible, non-toxic protein. With shellfish, take special care that these have grown in clean, unpolluted water a long way from a sewage outlet, as they are scavengers by nature!

Another idea is to go for wild game, but again be careful here because much game is reared by keepers to be hunted, and may also have been fed on chemically augmented food. If possible, check that it really is wild and not intensively reared.

Of course, the best source of genuinely organic eggs is to buy three or four hens and keep them yourself, if at all possible, as they should supply ample eggs for an average family.

IF I GO VEGAN, DO I NEED EXTRA VITAMIN B12?

Of particular concern is whether vegans get sufficient B12 to remain healthy – deficiency states can lead to anaemia. The answer to this is to make sure there is balance in your diet, particularly ensuring that you take in a good mixture of pulses, cereals, seeds and nuts every day, as well as a good cross-section of vegetables (including root vegetables as well as leafy vegetables and salads). If you are very concerned, you can easily supplement your intake with occasional fish or B12 in tablet form.

WILL I LOSE WEIGHT ON THIS DIET?

It is very likely that changing to a healthy diet will cause the loss of excess weight, which will be very welcome for most of us. This is because of the decrease in consumption of fat, protein, sugar and refined carbohydrate.

The problem comes, however, if the diet becomes too biased towards vegetable, salad and juice consumption with insufficient intake of carbohydrates such as bread, pasta, biscuits and cakes, rice, cereals and pulses. When first adopting this diet, there can be a tendency to eat almost exactly what somebody else might on a weight-loss diet. This is because many people have read about anti-cancer diets made up of mainly raw vegetables, and have inadvertently lost the balance in their diet. The solution is simple. Make sure that balance is achieved (this will be clarified later in this chapter, under Planning and Shopping). The main rule of thumb, however, is that if weight loss has become excessive, build up the carbohydrate element of the diet by increasing your intake of pasta, rice, potatoes and whole-food biscuits and cakes, and the fat element with oily dressings.

WILL CUTTING SALT OUT OF MY DIET CAUSE PROBLEMS, AS SALT IS ESSENTIAL FOR LIFE?

Almost every foodstuff we eat contains salt, and without adding a single grain of salt to anything we cook or eat, we will get adequate salt for our physiological requirements. The extensive use of salt in our cooking is solely to do with flavour and can really become quite addictive, with greater and greater amounts of salt being used. As with giving up sugar in tea or coffee, it is surprising how quickly we adjust and how quickly thereafter the taste of highly salted food is a real shock to the system.

One palpable benefit of reducing salt intake is a reduction of symptoms in those who have premenstrual syndrome and fluid retention. It would appear that the extra water retention experienced naturally towards the end of a menstrual cycle is exacerbated by the presence of a great deal of salt in the body, and this can tip susceptible individuals into irritability, depression and all the other symptoms of this syndrome.

Some people try to achieve a salt flavour in their diet with the use of potassium chloride (*LO-Salt*) instead of sodium chloride. While this is less harmful than sodium overload it still distorts the electrolyte balance within the body. It is far better to get used to the natural taste of foods if possible.

DO I NEED TO GIVE UP HONEY AS WELL AS SUGAR?

As explained in Chapter 1, it is important to wean ourselves off foods which contain large amounts of refined white sugar because of the stress this puts on our system, the obesity it creates, and the satisfaction it gives without conferring nutritional benefits. High sugar levels in the body also predispose us to infections and have been postulated to create conditions in which cancer cells may thrive.

Having said this, glucose (a simple form of sugar) is the final endpoint for all our metabolic pathways and the source of all our energy. As with salt, all our foods contain sugars. Augmenting our natural sugar intake in a restrained way with the judicious use of small amounts of honey will therefore do no harm. Honey (unlike refined sugar) also contains other nutrient factors such as vitamins and minerals which are extremely beneficial to health. Overall, therefore, the careful use of honey is not ill-advised if sweetening is required.

WHAT IF I CANNOT FIND OR AFFORD ORGANIC VEGETABLES OR FRUITS?

Try to go for fruit and vegetables that are as fresh as possible, locally grown and in season. Wash them very well and peel them if you know that sprays have been used. Buying local produce will at least mean that the foods are likely to have been left in the ground or on the tree until fully mature, as opposed to being ripened with gases on board ships in transport. It will also mean they will not have been covered in extra sprays for transportation purposes, or kept in cold storage for long periods with devitalizing effects on their enzymes. Again, if at all possible try growing what you can at home. Even if you can only manage a few rows of beetroot, turnip, lettuce or spinach, this will improve the quality and flavour of your food no end, and give you immense satisfaction into the bargain.

DO I NEED TO GIVE UP ALCOHOL?

Ideally, yes, or at least limit it to special occasions. Alcohol is very toxic to our systems, and is considered to cause five per cent of all cancers in the West. In some countries this figure rises to 12 per cent. Alcohol has a direct irritant effect on the tissues of the mouth, throat, oesophagus (gullet) and stomach. It also puts our whole system under strain, largely due to its intermediary metabolite acetaldehyde, which is what makes us feel so sick and tired after binge drinking. However, there are also other toxic factors within alcohol (particularly red wine) that can give us nasty headaches and hangovers.

There have been reports over the last 10 years that a glass of wine a day may help prevent arterial disease and extend life, but the evidence here relates to a combination of the relaxant effect of alcohol (which can be achieved in better ways by learning to relax directly) and the effect of the antioxidants found in the grapes. These can be found in all fruits, vegetables and fruit drinks without the hangover! So drinkers who comfort themselves with this message should take a harder look at the direct cancer risk associated with regular drinking and think again. The whole thrust of the change in diet in the prevention and treatment of cancer is to take the strain off the body, so clearly drinking any more than one or two glasses of wine or beer will begin to pull on the body's resources, whilst strong spirits will directly irritate the tissues.

Regrettably, for many people alcohol is such a key part of their way of life that to stop it altogether would constitute major deprivation. A good rule of thumb, then, is never to drink enough to give you a hangover, because the presence of a hangover means you have gone over into a toxic state. For most people, this means that a glass or two of wine, or a pint of beer, is within the allowable bounds. The other golden rule is to swap a greater volume of poor-quality alcohol for less of a higher quality, which is ideally organic.

Do I really need to give up stimulants such as caffeine, tobacco and 'recreational drugs'?

Almost every stimulant we use will put the body into a greater state of arousal. In these excited states we will burn up more energy which we may well need for our healing. As explained earlier, the state of arousal shifts the resources of the body away from the housekeeping functions into thinking-and-doing mode, which means that the maintenance work of healing and repair of tissues is compromised. Usually stimulants are used to help us escape how we are feeling. However, anything which causes us to go faster and bypass the normal signals of tiredness, hunger, sadness or depression means that we are failing to listen to the messages of our body and soul, and risk losing the integration and health of the system as a whole. It is far, far better to heed these messages – experience and express our emotions, and achieve our highs through the natural pleasures of love, communication, self-expression, creativity and sexuality.

However, as with unhealthy eating patterns, the habitual use of stimulants of any sort may well be masking an underlying emotional problem, and attempts to wean oneself off these substances usually requires having adequate support systems and counselling in place during the transition period.

It is comforting for those who love the experience of stimulants of one sort or another to know that all states which can be reached through stimulants can be attained through the practice of yoga, breath work and meditation. If the body did not have the receptors to react with the external stimulants, then they would have no effect on us. The receptors are there because the body itself makes similar substances which can give us these experiences naturally; an example of this is the discovery of the naturally occurring morphine within the brain called 'endorphin', which reacts with our own morphine receptors to relieve pain and give pleasure.

Through meditation, yoga and pranayama (breath work in yoga), altered states of consciousness can be reached, but when this is done naturally it is accompanied by an enormous sense of wellbeing, insight and self-love, as opposed to the chaos, danger, illegality and potential for overdose associated with the use of drugs and stimulants. Part of the danger is created because drugs produce mood/thought changes rapidly in a body and mind which may be completely unprepared, and in social situations which may be completely inappropriate. The body's own 'stimulants' will be secreted in appropriate response to the situation or the amount of disciplined inner work and exploration one has made.

WHY SHOULD I AVOID FOOD ADDITIVES?

Many food additives cause no problem whatsoever, but others have been found to be quite toxic, being implicated in cancer, behavioural disorders and allergy. The other problem is that many of them work by rendering the food inert and therefore less likely to rot. This compromises the vitality and nutritional benefit of the foods. In general, therefore, additives are best avoided if at all possible. This applies particularly to substances such as saltpetre (sodium nitrite) which is used for the curing of salami and meats, as this has been found to be carcinogenic. There is evidence from Japan that excessive intake of pickled foods is implicated in cancer of the oesophagus and stomach. In this case, rather like the irritation of smoking to the lungs, it can be seen that very vinegary or spicy food may directly irritate the mucous membrane lining of the gullet and stomach, causing cancer to develop.

Another problem is in the smoking of foods or cooking of foods with barbecues. This applies particularly to smoking fish and meat, and barbecuing hamburgers, sausages and meats. It has been discovered that the hydrocarbons in the smoke disrupt the fat and protein structure in foods, creating carcinogenic free radicals which can initiate the creation of tumours in the body. One study on the subject suggested that if we eat barbecued food we should really precede and follow our meal with vitamin C, betacarotene or vitamin E in order to deactivate the free radicals we have taken in![1] The subject of protecting ourselves with vitamins and minerals will be covered in Chapter 4.

HOW IMPORTANT IS THE QUALITY OF THE WATER I DRINK, AND HOW MUCH SHOULD I DRINK A DAY?

Good, clean, fresh water is one of the most vital constituents of a healthy diet. Our bodies are composed of more than 80 per cent water, and it is in the passage of water through our systems that all of the balancing, cleansing and excretory processes occur. Natural spring water contains minerals which are essential to life; it is also well oxygenated, tastes good and feels alive to drink. By contrast, a lot of our tap water tastes very chemical and may have an unpleasant 'used' whiff to it. Worse still, it may contain by-products of the petrochemical, agricultural and plastics industries. Water filters within the house will partly clean up tap water, but do not by and large clear the chlorine or organic pollutants out of the water. It is really a vexed question as we are so completely dependent on our drinking water, but water, like fat, is a universal solvent and readily takes up soluble chemicals.

The best solution is to find a natural spring close to your home from which you could collect water regularly (having had it checked for cleanness by your local environmental health unit). The second-best option is to buy genuine spring water; it is a good idea to get advice from *Which?* reports and Friends of the Earth as to which brands constitute the best-quality water available in the shops at any time.

The quality of our water is a matter of enormous importance and may yet be found to be a major factor in the increased cancer rates, particularly in hormonally-related cancers. In some reservoirs, male fish have been rendered infertile by the presence of by-products of the plastics industry which mimic oestrogen. It is up to all of us to lobby intensively for the cleaning up of our environment and water supply if we are to protect our health and the health of our children long term.

Once we have found a source of clean water, we should really be drinking around 2 litres (roughly 4 pints) per day. It is good to get ourselves back into the habit of drinking this as water rather than as squash, tea or coffee. This will be another good step in the process of detoxifying the body. Another idea is to try drinking water hot, especially in the mornings. This is helpful with elimination functions and is as comforting as the first cup of tea of the day, once you get used to it.

HOW MUCH RAW FOOD SHOULD I INCLUDE IN MY DIET?

Many of the successful anti-cancer diets revolve around the use of a great deal of raw fruit and vegetables and of vegetable and fruit juices. To follow healthy-eating guidelines for cancer prevention, the ideal is to have raw vegetables in the form of a salad with two meals per day, and raw fruit two to three times per day. This should be supplemented with home-made raw fruit or vegetable juice on a daily basis, if possible. The use of raw fruits and vegetables in juicing, 'spring cleaning' and detox or fasting diets will be discussed in Chapter 4. (Shop-bought juices are usually pasteurized which destroys the vital enzymes, making fresh, home-made juice infinitely better for you.)

WHAT ARE THE BEST DRINKS TO FORM PART OF A HEALTHY APPROACH TO NUTRITION?

The most important drinks to avoid are those containing high levels of sugar, colourings and additives. Most 'pop' or fizzy drinks fall into this category. These should be replaced with either pure fruit and vegetable juices (preferably home-made) or the ever-increasing wonderful selection of new carbonated fruit juice drinks which have been developed. If in doubt, consult the ingredients list on the bottle; do not buy any which have added sugars, colourings and/or flavourings. Gradually attempt to substitute tea and coffee with herbal teas and coffee substitutes. If you cannot give up tea and coffee altogether, choose the decaffeinated varieties for intermittent use.

Cooking Guidelines

COOKING METHODS

As mentioned earlier, some cooking methods have been found to create carcinogens in our food. The worst offenders are barbecuing and smoking of foods (especially meat and meat fats), and the overheating of fat in deep-frying processes (and particularly the repeated use of cooking oils; this produces dangerous free radicals which can be potentially cancer-causing). It is therefore advisable to keep clear of barbecued meats and to restrict frying to a minimum. When you do fry, always use clean oil and do not heat it until it smokes. Many foods can be 'fried' in a little water, and cold oil can be added at the end for flavour and texture. This technique is often described by Kenneth Lo in many of his wok recipes using sesame oil.

The best cooking methods to master are steaming, stir-frying, stewing, roasting or baking food. Steaming and stir-frying mean that foods can be cooked quickly and lightly, thereby retaining much of their natural texture and nutrients. Baking, roasting and stewing foods are gentler ways of cooking which allow flavours to melt into one another on the stove or in the oven. The other technique to master is the making of a great variety of salads incorporating many different vegetables, pulses, grains, fruits, nuts and seeds.

In the main, you are trying to cook fruit and vegetables for the minimum amount of time, to render them tender but retain their juices and nutrients. Flavours can be enhanced in a multitude of ways: with herbs, spices, vinegar, soy sauce and miso (a black bean paste).

Microwaving

The safety of microwaved food poses a real dilemma. We are reassured that it is totally safe, but during microwaving, very high-energy microwaves are put into the food, instantly causing rapid oscillation of the food molecules, and therefore very high heats. You will have noticed that if you try to eat something straight out of the microwave oven it is unnaturally hot in a very different way from food out of a conventional oven. We are supposed to leave microwaved food for a set 'stand time' after cooking in order to allow some of this very high energy to dissipate, but often we do not. This means that some of this high energy gets dispersed to the cells lining the gullet and stomach, which could have dangerous irritant effects.

There is also the consideration of what happens to the vitamins and enzymes within foods that are microwaved. We know they are destroyed by the high temperatures of frying and pressure cooking, and so again this does not bode well for foods heated so hot and so fast. There is also the more difficult consideration of what this blast of high energy does to the subtler energy or vital force of the food. So all in all it would appear safer to stick to traditional methods of cooking, or to use the microwave only minimally. At the very least, be extremely careful to follow the manufacturers' instructions about leaving food for the recommended 'stand times' before eating it.

KITCHEN EQUIPMENT

It can be extremely helpful to invest in a good food processor with shredding and grating attachments. In this way a coleslaw or mixed raw vegetable salad can be made in seconds. The food processor will also help in chopping and mixing nuts and other ingredients for nut roasts and vegetable pâtés.

Purchasing a juicer (ideally a juice press) is also very helpful, not only for making up vegetable and fruit juices but also for preparing vegetable juice to use as a basis for delicious sauces which can be thickened with cornflour or arrowroot and served with main meals. Juices also provide an excellent and quick basis for soups. Juiced or puréed vegetables can also be used to replace oil in a vinaigrette.

For steaming purposes it can be helpful to invest in a small steaming unit which you can fit into any saucepan. These resemble flowers, with 'petals' that open. They stand on three small legs about one inch off the bottom of the pan, and are made of metal with many perforations. The 'petals' can open to varying degrees according to the size of the pan. The flavour of vegetables steamed in this way is a complete revelation for those of us brought up on boiled vegetables, and of course you do not lose all the vitamins and minerals into the water as you do when boiling them. A variety of other types of steamers is available if you wish to steam larger quantities of food. The Chinese supermarket is often a good source of different types of steamers as the Chinese steam much of their food.

Another purchase you can make at the Chinese supermarket or kitchen shop is a good wok. A wok is essentially a frying pan but its gentle, curved shape makes it ideal for stir-frying vegetables, as you can keep tossing the contents of the pan gently to make sure all the vegetables get cooked evenly. Electric woks are also available but are less versatile as it is not so easy to toss vegetables in them.

It is also important to check that you have at least two good chopping boards (one for savoury and one for sweet) and some good knives – some people like to chop their vegetables with a Chinese chopping knife, which is very fast and sharp. Basically, you will need at least one good, strong, longish knife, a small vegetable and herb-cutting knife, and a small mandolin-style vegetable peeler (which peels vegetables much more rapidly than the standard peeler). It is also helpful to have a pestle and mortar for crushing spices, and a garlic press. A nice refinement is to have a clean coffee grinder for the grinding of seeds, nuts and spices for certain recipes, but this is by no means essential. While it is good to experiment fully with all the herbs and flavours available, it is wise not to get hooked on using too many strong spices, pickles or chillies, as these can irritate the gut lining and are thought in some cultures to promote the development of cancer in the gut. The other requirements – such as casserole dishes, pans, wooden spoons – form part of the equipment of any normal kitchen.

Food Review

Now is the moment to introduce you to the huge choice of foods you have at your disposal once you start to feed yourself in a healthy way.

BREAKFAST CEREALS

The king of the breakfast cereals has to be muesli. Traditionally, this is made from a mixture of four or five different flakes, such as wheat, barley, rye and oats, with a combination of fruit such as raisins, sultanas and dates, and of nuts such as hazelnuts or cashews. Most health-food shops now stock at least four or five types of muesli which are augmented with other things such as coconut, apricots, sunflower seeds, pumpkin seeds, crystallized pineapple, dried apricots and figs. You can choose either to buy one of these or to buy a basic muesli and augment it yourself with goodies to suit your own taste.

It is good to try to develop a taste for muesli with either soya milk, rice milk or fruit juice. It is particularly good if soaked in one of these overnight, as the dried fruit plumps up and becomes quite delicious. It is also good to put fresh fruit such as apple, banana and/or grapes onto muesli for a really satisfying breakfast.

There is also a crunchier type of muesli called granola. This is made from cereals which have been coated with honey and toasted, and is quite delicious. A recipe for Crunchy Granola Breakfast Cereal can be found in Chapter 5.

We have all heard of cornflakes, but it is also possible to get wheat flakes, rice flakes, buckwheat flakes, millet flakes and barley flakes. Some wheat flakes can be coated in malt or honey, and you can also experiment with puffed rice cereal and puffed wheat. In specialist whole-food shops you may find a delicious breakfast cereal called *Kashi*, which is a mixture of seven puffed whole grains and sesame.

Another lovely discovery is jumbo oats, which make a really satisfying porridge. They are bigger than ordinary porridge oats and have much more texture and flavour. They are also delicious in many dessert and biscuit recipes. Of course it is also fun to experiment with the traditional oatmeal porridges, and for this purpose it is quite wise to invest in a slow overnight porridge cooker, unless you have an Aga with a slow oven, and to buy good-quality organic oatmeal. You can also experiment with other grains to make porridge, such as millet, brown rice, wheat flakes, rice flakes or even buckwheat. Again, you will find excellent porridge recipes in the 'Breakfasts' section in Chapter 5.

BREAKFAST FRUITS

A really lovely way to start the day is with a fruit compote. Most dried fruits are sweet enough to make a beautiful syrup with the addition of water or fruit juice alone, and lightly stewed prunes, figs, apricots or a mixture of dried apples and pears make a really delicious breakfast. There is a wonderful dried apricot called the hunza apricot. It is particularly delicious if you stand it for 24 hours covered in water to which has been added a bay leaf and a few cardamom seeds. You then bring it to the boil and simmer it gently for just 5 minutes, then leave it to stand in the juice for another 24 hours. It is a really luxurious dessert, especially with a soya or nut cream.

The other thing to do with fruit is to have a lovely fresh fruit salad. This also makes a particularly satisfying breakfast. Alternatively, mix soaked dried fruit with the fresh fruit. As a substitute for yoghurt, try soya yoghurts and desserts. These are extremely good alternatives to their dairy counterparts and go very well with fruit compotes, fruit salads or muesli.

BREADS

Thankfully, the age of bread has really come again, and most bakers, delicatessens, supermarkets and health-food shops have a truly wonderful selection of whole-food breads. I recommend you try three-seed bread, which has a mixture of sunflower, sesame and poppy seeds; granary bread, which includes whole-wheat grains; wholemeal bread or, better still, organic wholemeal. This tends to be less light than the bread we are used to, but is extremely tasty and packed with goodness. It is also possible to get a selection of Italian and Indian breads containing herbs, sun-dried tomatoes, olives and spices; these can add wonderful variety to your meals. Speciality bakers will also have breads made from rye, barley or rice flours as well as malted breads and fruited breads, which again make a delicious change. It is also possible to get whole-wheat teacakes and hot-cross buns, which are good for breakfast as well as tea!

Fruit spreads and honey

There is an astounding selection of honeys available from good health-food stores, from the delicately flavoured acacia honey to more robust, tangy buckwheat – from the creamy white clover honey to the dark Greek mountain honey, and the very sweet, translucent orange blossom honeys. Ideally, you should get organic honey from bees which have not been sugar-fed. You should use honey in moderation such as on toast or in tea, and not in huge quantities as a pure sugar substitute.

As an alternative to honey there is malt syrup, rice syrup, corn and barley syrups, as well as pure malt extract. An interesting change is date syrup or molasses, each of which has its own very specific flavour, and of course there is maple syrup. This variety drives home the fact that so many foods contain natural sugars and it is fun to experiment with all the different flavours – again in moderation.

The area of fruit spreads is another joy to explore, and these can be used for preserves and cakes as well as on toast at breakfast. In many shops, and particularly health-food shops, you can find a wonderful selection of sugar-free jams, including apricot, cherry, blackberry and apple, blackcurrant, strawberry and raspberry, as well as the more exotic varieties such as guava and mango conserve, banana and mango spread, pineapple and ginger spread, and peach and passion fruit spread! You will also find a dark, thick spread called pear and apple spread, made by Sun Wheel, which is not the texture of ordinary jam but more like a dark paste. This is quite delicious, and Whole Earth also make a pear and apricot spread. It is also possible to get low-sugar marmalade, and so toast and marmalade is definitely still on the menu!

Drinks

I have suggested trying to cut out tea and coffee because of their stimulant properties, but if you are unable to do this altogether then you could try a brand called *Luaka*, a very pleasant decaffeinated tea. It is also possible to get Twinings decaffeinated Earl Grey tea in major supermarkets. Decaffeinated coffee is available both in instant form and as coffee beans. There are those who say that the process of decaffeination renders coffee more toxic than it is in its natural form, and that it may be better to have the occasional cup of 'whole' coffee than to have decaffeinated coffee regularly.

By and large it is better to develop a taste for herbal teas and tisanes, and again there is a startling variety. The traditional herbal teas are made from herbs, as the name suggests, the classic ones being camomile, peppermint, elderflower, hibiscus, lemon verbena, lime flower and fennel. However, the 1970s and 1980s saw an absolute burgeoning in the area of fruit teas, and you can get anything from lemon zinger, country peach passion, wild forest blackberry, Mediterranean citrus or mixed fruit and rosehip to pineapple and coconut or passion fruit vanilla! There are many other varieties too, and they are nice chilled as well as hot. It is great in the summer to make up a big pot of herbal tea and then strain it and keep it in a jug in the fridge. The addition of some ice, fresh herbs (particularly mint) and a slice or two of fresh fruit makes an extremely refreshing and healthy alternative to cordials or sweetened drinks.

Another idea, if you are very fond of tea, is to move to a much more delicate type of tea such as jasmine, green or china tea, which can be drunk very weak without milk or perhaps with a slice of lemon. There is also the very distinctive and unusual Japanese twig or *bancha* tea, which is said to have anti-cancer properties. This is made by boiling twigs and then sieving or straining the liquid to drink. It is quite delicious and brings with it shades of the Japanese tea ritual. Green tea also has direct anti-cancer properties. Other unusual varieties of tea are *Mu* tea and *Rooibosch* tea; the latter is made from the African red bush and has a very distinctive, tangy tea flavour and far less tannin or stimulants. Of course, with tea it is not just the caffeine we have to think about, but the bitter acidity of the tannin. If you try drinking your normal strength of tea without any milk in it you will be surprised at just how bitter it is, and many of us are subjecting our systems to this acid brew nine or more times a day!

There are many other healthy drinks which are sometimes used as coffee substitutes. However, I prefer to see them as drinks in their own right, not as coffee substitutes, as this does not create a false sense of expectation (none of them really tastes like coffee at all!). There is *Barleycup*, made from roasted barley, and *Yannoh* and *Bambu*, which are made from a mixture of grains, herbs and figs. There is also dandelion coffee made from roasted dandelion roots (which is a little more bitter), as well as the more chocolatey carob-based drinks which, if anything, resemble the taste of cocoa.

Juices

Juices come in all shapes and sizes, though the older-style cartoned juices most commonly available in supermarkets tend to be of a rather poor quality. This is because the juice is usually 'concentrated' (that is, most of the liquid evaporated off) in the country of origin, shipped in this concentrated form, and then diluted again for sale in the destination country. In this process many of the nutrients, particularly the vitamins and enzymes, will have been damaged. Again, it is better to get organic, whole, locally produced juice if you can. The best juice in Britain is, therefore, that made from apples, as we grow so many. A fresh organic apple juice will taste every bit as good as a fresh crunchy apple. Many supermarkets and juice bars now sell freshly squeezed juices individually or as delicious mixtures. As long as these have not been pasteurized they form an absolutely ideal anti-cancer drink. Good brands are *P and J* or *Innocents*, and many supermarkets also have their own brand of fresh juice.

Unfortunately, many cartoned or bottled vegetable juices have by law to be pasteurized. This is understandable because of potential bacterial contamination from the earth, but the process is likely to affect the juice's nutrient content. The best solution is to buy your own juicer, scrub your organic vegetables clean, and make up mixtures of fruits and vegetables, such as beetroot, carrot and apple, to create your own absolutely delicious fresh juices. Of course, when you first get your juicer, most things in your kitchen will go into it as you experiment with everything from potatoes to turnips, celery and bananas! The bizarre thing with bananas is that they produce hardly any juice, though if you put a banana through the juicer and follow up with other fruits, the resulting juice will have a wonderful banana flavour. It is also possible to use the fibrous waste products from the juicing process to make a vegetable stockpot. In this way you will feel very virtuous as you squeeze the last scrap of goodness out of your organic vegetables! Ideally, remember to peel and discard the skin of non-organic vegetables and fruits before you put them in the juicer, as these can contain alarmingly high levels of pesticides and insecticides.

The New Drinks

Since people have cottoned on to the fact that taking in large amounts of sugar in canned drinks is a bad idea for our teeth, metabolism, weight and nutrition, a whole new spectrum of drinks has evolved. These usually take the form of fruit juice concentrates diluted with sparkling mineral water. The first really successful brand was *Aqua Libra*, which has a refreshing melon-like flavour; this was closely followed by elderflower drinks, apple drinks and other mixed fruit drinks.

There is also a selection of fruit juice concentrates available such as apple, pear, strawberry, blackcurrant and many more. Because these have all been heated in order to be concentrated, again they are not so good nutritionally but they do make wonderful natural flavourings for healthy desserts such as mousses and whips made with soya products. They can also be used to flavour the syrups in fruit salad, or to add interesting flavours to a sweet-and-sour sauce. Concentrates can also be used in place of sweeteners, because, being so concentrated, they are really quite sweet.

By far the best drink of all is good-quality water. As mentioned earlier, if you can find a spring, get the water quality checked and then regularly fetch yourself some fresh spring water, as it is absolutely the ideal water to drink. Failing this rather idyllic possibility, seek out the best-quality bottled water you can find, and try to drink around 2 litres (4 pints) a day, either cold or in herbal teas and tisanes.

PULSES

For most of us the image of pulses stops with red and green lentils, red kidney beans and dried peas! If this is the case for you, prepare to be very pleasantly surprised; this at first intimidating area of whole-food cookery will soon become a great delight. Pulses will become one of your main sources of protein if you choose to follow this diet, so it is important to work your way through any nervousness you have about cooking them so that you can really benefit from the wonderful variety of textures and flavours that are available. In the meantime, as you start to acquire these new skills you will be happy to know that many pulses are now available precooked in tins in the supermarket. While it is healthier and often more rewarding to cook beans fresh, there are occasions when convenience is most important.

Lentils

I did not mean to mock the red lentil – it is an extremely useful food which can be used to make delicious soups and Indian dahl, and forms the solid element in many roasts and bakes. Presently much more fashionable are the green puy lentils which have a delicious flavour and do not become as mushy as the red kind when cooked up. Nice alternatives are ordinary brown or green lentils, and if you go into an Indian store you will find an incredible array of between 10 and 20 other types of lentils to experiment with. The Indian shopkeepers will happily tell you how to cook the different varieties; literally every time I have asked for advice I have been invited to the shopkeeper's home to be shown in person! The Indians, especially the Hindus, are usually wonderful vegetable cooks and they also have a stunningly generous attitude to food and its preparation. Following up on such an invitation can lead you into a real adventure, and may well end up in a long-term, highly educational friendship!

Peas

The pea family is also quite large. As well as the dried green pea, which forms the basis of England's beloved 'mushy peas', there are chickpeas (sometimes known as garbanzo beans), which can be used in stews, salads and also as the basis of the delicious Greek dish known as hummus. This is made from chickpeas, garlic, olive oil, lemon juice and tahini, and makes an extremely tasty dip or spread. There are also green and yellow split peas, most commonly found in soup recipes.

Beans

One of the finest and tastiest gourmet beans is the flageolet. This is smaller than a red kidney bean, is light green in colour and has a delicate flavour. The other rather fine bean is the aduki bean, which is small and dark red and has a very rich flavour. Black kidney beans are rather like red kidney beans only a little smaller, and there is even another similar bean called a black turtle bean which comes from the US. These are both quite distinct from the small, very highly flavoured Chinese black bean, used to enrich sauces, fish and vegetable dishes and to make miso pastes for flavouring soups and stews. Black-eyed beans are different again: they are rather small white/tan beans with a little 'black eye' at one end where the bean adjoins the pod. Again, these are great for bean stews.

The large white butter bean is one of my favourites – it is wonderful to sauté cooked butter beans gently in olive oil, garlic and parsley, or to purée them as the basis for a dip or pâté. They also make wonderful soups and stews as they have such a rich, distinctive flavour. Cannellini beans are white and slightly smaller than red kidney beans, and form a very suitable main course bean. Field beans are round and brown and come from the UK, and take quite a lot of cooking. They are unusual and can add variety to your meal plans. Haricot beans are the ones used in tinned baked beans. In their natural state they are white; because they have such a lovely texture when cooked, they are again ideal for soups and stews. Mung beans are small and green and often used for sprouting purposes, producing the bean sprouts so commonly available at Chinese restaurants. Pinto beans are rather pink and speckled, and again form a slightly unusual alternative.

The red kidney bean is most commonly known for its use in Mexican chilli dishes. Happily, it is just as easy to make a chilli *sin carne* (without meat) as a chilli *con carne*; for most people starting out into vegan country this is a very easy recipe to master if you already know how to make chilli with minced beef. Some people keep, in fact, very close to the original recipe by substituting vegetarian mince products for minced beef (these will be described in detail later), but it is just as good to use beans alone. Red kidney beans also make a wonderful bean salad. Simply chop some onions, tomatoes, parsley and a little garlic, mix this with cold precooked beans in a good vinaigrette and you have a lovely starter or main course salad.

This brings us to the most astounding bean of all: the soya bean. It is hardly ever cooked and served as a bean, but is instead the basis for a most amazing range of products. This includes soya milk, bean curd (or tofu), soya yoghurt and desserts, soya cream, soya cheese and many other soya pastes and pâtés, meat substitutes, and even soya ice cream! Babies can be reared extremely well on soya milk instead of cow's milk formula, and this is often the solution to lactose intolerance and the type of eczema/asthma associated with cow's milk and dairy foods. The soya bean is a small white bean which takes a lot of cooking to eat as a bean. To make milk it is simply ground and diluted with water. Like cow's-milk, this will then set to make yoghurt and bean curd, and the curd can be pressed just like cow's-milk curd to make cheeses and more dense pâtés and pastes, which can be used in a variety of ways. Much of the vegetarian pre-prepared food sold in the supermarket is based upon soya.

RICE, GRAINS AND PASTA

The starch component of our meals is the part that provides the main energy source, as starch is easily converted into glucose for fuelling our bodies. In the British diet the potato has long been the staple starchy food, while in most other parts of the world, especially Third World countries, the staple starch source comes from rice and grains. Rice and grains are far higher in vitamins and minerals than potatoes. They are particularly high in the B and E vitamins, essential fatty acids, vegetable protein and minerals (provided they have been grown in a good-quality soil). In fact, it has even been mooted that potatoes were introduced as the staple diet of peasants in the Middle Ages because it kept them less intelligent than if they were fed on a grain-based diet!

Many of the vitamins and minerals contained in potatoes and other root vegetables are concentrated 2mm under their skins, and very often the skins are discarded. The same is true of rice and grains, and so it is important to go for whole grains – such as brown rice rather than white. Unpeeled scrubbed potatoes, boiled or cooked in their skins, are delicious and very wholesome (if organic). In general, however, the aim is to eat at least one meal per day using rice and grains as the key element.

Rice

With rice, the main choice you have is between long-grain and short-grain brown rice. Arborio rice, which comes from Italy, makes fantastic risottos and the rather finer brown rice, which comes from Pakistan, is called basmati rice.

Short-grain brown rice is not just for puddings (as is short-grain white rice); it just tends to have a slightly stickier quality when cooked than the lighter long-grain brown rice. This makes it a good choice for risottos, whereas I would recommend long-grain rice for a salad where it is more important that the grains remain separate and do not become at all stodgy.

For a real treat there is also a wonderful rice known as wild rice, which commonly comes from Surinam. This looks completely different, being much finer and longer than ordinary rice, and being encased in a black shell. During cooking, the shells burst open and the rice swells, contrasting the white rice with the dark shell. The end result is very attractive, tasty and textured.

To cook most types of brown rice, one foolproof recipe is first to wash the rice and then add one-and-a-half mugs of water per mug of rice and simmer very gently until all the water is gone. Another method is to put a little oil in the pan first, heat it, add the rice and stir it round in the oil, making sure all the grains get covered, then add the water, bring it to the boil and simmer. This method has the added advantage of flavouring the rice nicely with a hint of sesame or olive oil. Either method should leave you with a perfect result. No salt is added during cooking, and usually a lid is left on the pan at a tilt to allow for slow evaporation of the water. This usually takes 30–40 minutes. The end result usually tastes great just as it is, though you can also flavour it with olive oil, linseed oil, roasted sesame seeds or a little soy sauce. It may also be flavoured by the addition of either 2–3 bay leaves or 6–8 cardamom pods while cooking. Wild rice usually takes a little longer to cook; most packets of wild rice come with good instructions. Sometimes a little precooked wild rice can be cooked separately and mixed with ordinary brown rice to add a little glamour.

If you are planning to make a rice salad, it can be a good idea to add your vinaigrette straight after cooking the rice, while the rice is cooling (having been drained of water), as this will keep the grains separate and the heat will help the flavour of the vinaigrette to be fully absorbed into the rice. Then, once the rice has cooled, it can be stored in the fridge in this way for later use, mixed with chopped vegetables, fruits, nuts and seeds. If you are intending to reheat the rice later to use in a savoury dish, then a small amount of olive oil added while cooling will help the rice grains stay separate and reheat easily.

A range of rice dishes can be found in Chapter 5, but to expand your knowledge of rice cookery and your repertoire of delicious recipes, I would strongly recommend that you study an Italian vegetarian cookery book to become familiar with the techniques used in cooking risottos, and Indian vegetarian cookery books for good recipes for pilau and biriani rice dishes.

Rice milk is an interesting alternative to soya milk. It is slightly less powdery in taste, and is therefore less likely to be noticed when used as a substitute for cow's milk.

Grains

If you are thinking that you are rapidly going to become bored with eating brown rice every day, do not worry: there is a wide selection of other grains to experiment with, some of which also have the advantage of cooking much more quickly than brown rice.

Wholemeal couscous is the first example that springs to mind. Couscous is made from wheat and takes only 20–30 minutes to cook. It can be used either as an accompaniment to vegetables or, like risotto, mixed with vegetables to make a main meal in its own right. Bulgar is also made from wheat, but has rather more texture and flavour than couscous. Both couscous and bulgar are used extensively in Middle Eastern dishes.

Quite different again is the flavour and texture of buckwheat. Buckwheat has a fairly strong flavour, which makes for an extremely interesting change. Its taste is enhanced even more by pre-roasting the buckwheat prior to boiling it. In fact, all grains respond well to pre-roasting or toasting in a pan prior to boiling.

Another wonderful grain is pearl barley, which has a lovely texture and flavour and originates from the UK. We are perhaps most familiar with its use in soups, to thicken and enrich a winter vegetable broth, or perhaps in its other common use in the making of barley water. Traditionally, barley water had lemon and sugar added to it and was often given to invalids as a restorative. In fact, on its own, without the lemon and sugar, barley water is quite alkaline and can be a great help in the natural treatment of cystitis. My main point here is that it can also be used very effectively as a grain in its own right as an alternative to rice, and again cooks more quickly than rice.

There are other whole grains which can be used exactly as they are, such as wheat, rye, oats and millet. The more you experiment with these different grains, the more you will come to love their subtle and unique flavours and textures.

Another unusual grain is quinoa, which comes from Ecuador. This grain is particularly interesting as it contains all 22 essential amino acids – and is quite delicious. Finally, and highest on the list for entertainment value, is the grain made from maize – alias popcorn! Making your own popcorn is a riot and only requires a deep pan with a lid and a tiny bit of hot oil. You can render small children helpless with delight by putting far too much popcorn into the pan in one go, heating it up until it all starts to explode, calling them over to have a look, and then taking the lid off – which will end up with a fountain of popcorn shooting all over the kitchen, and your fun rating going up by at least 400 per cent.

Flours

Flours are made out of all the grains described above, and more things besides! Of course, where good organic, varied wholemeal flours come into their own is in the making of bread. It may be that, as with many people who have returned to this more natural, balanced way of eating, you get a strong urge to experiment with making your own bread. This has to be one of the most deeply satisfying forms of cooking, which brings with it a great sense of wellbeing and homeliness to all around you. It is a marvellous symbol of your intention to love and nurture yourself, and I recommend it wholeheartedly. It is wise to start with organic wholemeal flours, but if you progress and become more adventurous, you could experiment with mixtures, including barley and rye flours.

There is also, of course, cornflour, which is ideal for thickening sauces, and gram flour (made from chickpeas), which is wonderful for making very light, crisp batters. It is often used in Indian cookery for this purpose. There are also brown rice flours, soya flour and even potato flour and buckwheat flour, which you will find in some recipes but probably not often enough to merit their storage in your kitchen.

Pasta

Pasta is another good way to get your starchy staple into a meal. Strictly speaking, it is a processed food and will therefore be slightly less nutritious than the grains in their whole form. None the less, for most of us it is a realistic and appealing way to cook and eat carbohydrates. As well as appearing in a multitude of forms, it can also be made from the full spectrum of grains. Again, the golden rule is to go for brown rather than white pastas and to experiment with the different types to avoid becoming bored.

It is quite possible to get fusilli, lasagne, macaroni, penne, spaghetti, fettucini, tortellini, tagliatelle, shells and noodles in brown wheat pastas, and many of these different forms are also available in pastas made from buckwheat, corn and rice. Another interesting variation is pasta made from spelt, an Eastern European grain. It has a nutty flavour and is quite delicious.

Superior wheat pasta is made from the very hard durum wheat, which has a high gluten content and an extremely good flavour. Nowadays it is also possible to get many pastas which are already enriched with herbs, garlic, vegetables, chilli and even soya. Where soya has been mixed in, this will of course mean you are getting your carbohydrates and proteins at the same time.

Pastas can be used in hundreds of different ways, with sauces, in salads, in bakes and as noodles in soups (most commonly found in Chinese cooking). The best advice here is to get hold of an Italian vegetarian cookery book. Once you tune in to the many different uses of fresh herbs, mushrooms, tomatoes, nuts and seeds, you will never look back! Nowadays there is also a wide range of extremely good vegan precooked vegetable, tomato and mushroom pasta sauces for sale in supermarkets, which will be a great help for those with a busy lifestyle.

Nuts and seeds

The use of nuts by the British seems to be confined to the purchasing of a large quantity for Christmas, which then lies around gathering dust until the summer (when they are finally, begrudgingly, thrown in the bin!), or the consumption of extremely salty peanuts in bars and pubs. Seeds, for their part, do not really feature in the average Western diet at all. In both cases this is a great shame, because nuts and seeds form an invaluable source of protein, vitamins, minerals and essential fatty acids as well as being wonderfully varied in their flavours, textures and potential uses.

Nuts

The first thing to be aware of with nuts is the extraordinary difference between fresh nuts and nuts which have been hanging around for a long time in our shops and cupboards. Fresh nuts are usually soft and sweet with quite a creamy texture, whereas old nuts tend to become more brittle, bitter and increasingly rancid.

Needless to say, it is important to try to get hold of nuts that are in season and as fresh as possible.

The most useful nuts in whole-food cooking are cashews, almonds, brazils, hazelnuts, walnuts, macadamia nuts and pecans. An absolutely delicious contribution from the nut and seed world can be made by the addition of pistachios and pine kernels to your cooking and salads. In fact, both of these are so tasty that I would not be surprised if they never make it into the cooking pot at all!

Nuts can be used to form the basis of a roast or bake, which can be flavoured with curry spices, herbs or left plain for the natural flavours of the nuts to emerge fully. Nut roasts can be eaten hot or cold, and can be a wonderful substitute for the meat component of a meal. They can be accompanied by a sauce, perhaps made from tomatoes or vegetable juices, as the only criticism of a nut roast is that it can sometimes be rather dense and rich.

A little further along this spectrum, nuts can be used to make pâtés mixed with other ingredients, and of course puréed or processed in their own right to make savoury or sweet spreads. For example, hazelnuts, pecans, peanuts and almonds are all available as nut butters, whereas puréed cashew nuts, with the addition of a little soya milk and apple juice, make an absolutely wonderful cream topping for desserts.

Nuts, especially when fresh, can be curried with absolutely wonderful results. They can also be roasted either on their own or with a little soy sauce added to enhance their flavour, either to eat as they are or mix into salads, or for use as toppings on baked dishes. They can be mixed into rice dishes, pasta dishes and vegetable stuffings. Whole chestnuts can become a delightful focus for a stew, or are absolutely brilliant puréed as the central ingredient in vegetable bakes and vegetable stuffings. Chestnut purée can be used sweetened with fruit syrups as the basis for many whole-food desserts and cake fillings.

Nut butters mixed with carob have a flavour similar to chocolate and are great for tempting children. Carob is used in preference to chocolate as it does not contain caffeine or other stimulants. Coconut is another extremely versatile nut. Like chestnuts, creamed coconut can make a wonderful addition to a curry or vegetable bake, and serves equally well as a basis for desserts and cakes. Coconut also toasts beautifully in flakes for toppings which can be used on both savoury and sweet dishes. Coconut milk is, of course, also available and equally versatile. Coconut cream is made from the puréed flesh of the coconut and can be used to great effect in drinks. For example, coconut cream mixed with pineapple juice, crushed ice and fresh lime makes a wonderfully refreshing fruit cocktail; the addition of rum to this mixture creates the delicious *bahia* of the Far East. Overall, however, you should use coconut in moderation as it contains saturated fats, which have been linked with arterial disease.

Seeds

It is not really surprising that seeds should have such a high nutritional value. They contain within them all the essentials for the creation of a new plant. In fact, the sprouting of seeds is another way in which their nutritional potential can be released and enhanced, as the sprouts become very rich in plant enzymes as well as the vitamins, minerals, proteins and essential fatty acids contained in the seeds themselves.

Seeds tend to be used either whole, plain or roasted, or ground into pastes, powders or spreads. Many have such a high oil content that extraction of this oil becomes the main commercial use of these seeds. The most popular seeds for whole-food cookery are sunflower, sesame, linseed, alfalfa and pumpkin seeds. When ground in a specially designated coffee grinder, they can be sprinkled onto sweet and savoury dishes to enhance the flavour and nutritional value. They are also delicious mixed with sliced fresh fruit, soya yoghurt, vanilla and honey or maple syrup.

Sunflower Seeds

Sunflower seeds can be used whole in bakes, stuffings and toppings, and are particularly delicious roasted in the oven after tossing lightly in shoyu or soy sauce. This way they can be used as a good pre-dinner snack with drinks, or to go into children's lunch boxes.

Sesame Seeds

Sesame seeds are tiny and extremely tasty. They are wonderful for adding texture and flavour to pastries, breads and savoury crumble toppings. Ground into a paste, they form the delicious savoury spread known as *tahini*, which comes in light and dark forms. Tahini is used extensively in Middle Eastern cookery and is a very useful addition to vegetable stews (to add texture and flavour), as a side sauce with rice and vegetables, or quite simply on a piece of toast with margarine, topped for garlic lovers with a quarter of a clove of crushed garlic! It also forms the basis for the delicious Greek and Middle Eastern sweet called *halva*, which will be described in the section on 'Snacks and Sweets'. They can also be roasted with a little sea salt and ground to form *gomasio*, which is described in the section on flavouring.

Pumpkin Seeds

Pumpkin seeds are large and oval-shaped with pointed ends. They are sometimes added to muesli and bakes and are absolutely delicious when roasted with a little soy sauce until brown.

Alfalfa Seeds

Alfalfa seeds are absolutely tiny and can be added to foods for their nutrient value, or used for sprouting the very fine, delicate sprouts which are now sometimes available in supermarkets and health-food stores. This is a great relief for many of us who have ended up with rather smelly variations on a theme of our third-form biology class on the window sills of our kitchens – I certainly take my hat off to those who can effortlessly produce crunchy, delicious sprouts at home. No matter how you obtain them, alfalfa sprouts – along with the mung bean sprouts mentioned earlier – make a wonderful nutritious addition to salads and stir-fried vegetables.

The other seed you may well come across is the blue poppy seed, which has a fine flavour and a beautiful appearance and can be used in a variety of sweet and savoury dishes.

Linseed

Linseed, as mentioned earlier, is becoming increasingly used as a supplemental source of omega-3 fatty acids, and can easily be incorporated, ground, into many dishes.

OILS AND MARGARINES

Oils

Oils can be produced from a wonderful variety of nuts and seeds. In the 1940s, 1950s and 1960s, along with the tendency to refine all other types of foods, oils were produced in such a refined state that it was hardly possible to distinguish the taste of the nut or seed of origin. Now, thankfully, there has been a return to natural cold-pressed virgin oils which retain both their natural flavouring and colouring. There is no comparison whatsoever between the delicious dark green virgin olive oil, dark brown walnut or hazelnut oils, or deep golden peanut oil with their insipid, pale yellow, refined counterparts. A small dash of pure sesame oil added at the end of a stir-fry dish can give a wonderful depth of flavour, and the nut oils are excellent for flavouring vinaigrettes. Peanut oil is particularly good for Chinese cooking. Soya oil, sunflower oil, corn oil and safflower oil are less fully flavoured, but are cheap and wholesome. Almond, coconut and grape seed oil are rather more delicate and are sometimes used in cake recipes. Mustard oil, however, is not used in food at all, as it has a very high erucic acid content. Ghee, which is often found in Indian shops, is usually made from butter and as such is best avoided. However, some whole-food shops sell a vegetable form of ghee. In the main, olive oil substitutes well for ghee in Indian recipes.

Margarines

There is now a plethora of margarines available on the market, but actually very few of these are vegan. Most contain some form of milk solids and are best avoided (even many of the new olive-oil margarines contain milk solids). It is best to look carefully at the list of ingredients on the label. Two of the healthiest vegan margarines sold in the UK are *Vitaquel* and *Granose*.

SOYA PRODUCTS

It has already been mentioned that the soya bean produces the most fantastic range of products, which is even more fortuitous now that soya is considered to be so beneficial. One of the first enormously helpful things for the vegan is the way that soya can be used to replace most dairy products. Soya milk tastes slightly chalky compared to cow's milk, but goes well with tea and on breakfast cereals. (It does not work, however, with coffee, as it seems to curdle.) Soya cream is remarkably good, and soya yoghurts – particularly if flavoured with fresh fruit – are an excellent substitute.

If you find it impossible to give up all milk-based yoghurt completely, goat's-milk yoghurt is by far the best as it is low-fat and the proteins are very easily digestible. Sheep's yoghurt, however, is even creamier than most cow's-milk yoghurts. For example, much of the creamy Greek yoghurt sold is made from sheep's milk. Soya cheese is perhaps the least good of the substitutes and may not really be worth including in your diet.

Soya beans are also fermented and made into an extremely good flavouring paste called *miso*, which makes an excellent replacement for the stock cube and will be described later (in the section on 'Spices and Flavourings').

The next stage along the soya path is into tofu territory. Tofu is a soft, rather jelly-like light curd made from soya milk left to stand and separate like curds and whey. The curd is pressed into square blocks which can be bought in brine from health-food shops and Chinese supermarkets. This is what the Chinese call 'bean curd', and it can be used in a variety of ways. When it is incorporated into other dishes it is best to simmer it for a few minutes first to make it slightly more solid, otherwise it will crumble if stirred into sauces or vegetable dishes. It soaks up other flavours well, which is good because it is actually very mildly flavoured itself. Tofu can also be fried, which gives it a light brown, crispy coating. Skilled cooks can manage to stuff tofu with piquant sauces and vegetable mixtures and fry this to produce a mouth-watering snack or starter. There is a very light form of tofu called 'silken tofu', which can be used as a base for making quiches and cheesecake. Silken tofu can also be used as a base for vegan milkshakes and build-up drinks.

Tofu is also used mixed with other ingredients to form the base of many savoury whole-food products such as burgers, pâtés, pasty fillings and bakes. Apart from soya yoghurt, on the dessert front it is also possible to buy soya desserts made by *Provamel*, *Lima* and *Sojasun*, which come in vanilla, banana and carob flavours. These are rather like mousse or custard, and are ideal desserts for children or as toppings on fruits and other puddings. Somehow they seem to be less chalky than most soya yoghurts, and children take to them very readily.

Meat alternatives

There has been an extraordinary development in the past 20 years of a whole range of vegetarian meat substitutes, due to the burgeoning of vegetarianism. By and large, these products are made out of textured vegetable protein (TVP) or Quorn, which is made from a myco-protein. This myco-protein, which has an extremely good nutritional profile (being very low in fat and very high in all the essential amino acids), was originally found growing underground in the Thames Valley and is now grown commercially in specially designed plants. TVP and Quorn can be made into a whole variety of meat substitutes because their texture is rather chewy, like that of meat. Quorn is slightly firmer than TVP, so a little closer to meat in texture. They do not naturally have a very strong flavour, but, like tofu, take on very well the flavours of sauces and marinades. TVP and Quorn can be bought as 'mince', 'chunks' (which represent stewing steak), or paste, which can be made up into sausages and burgers.

This is fantastically helpful for those who find that they wish to adopt a vegan or vegetarian diet without changing the type of meals that they eat. To help us even further there is now an increasingly good range of products on the market, with items such as meatless shepherd's pie, non-meat meat pies and vegan sausage rolls, which would easily deceive the average meat-eater if only for the joyous fact that you never come across any offending bits of gristle or tubes! The only snag with this approach is that it may tend to keep you locked into the practice of basing your meals around large amounts of protein, but as long as you bear in mind the intention to reduce your protein intake to around 10–20 per cent of the meal, this is fine.

BISCUITS

Happily, many savoury biscuits are already made from whole-food ingredients. For example, oatcakes are an absolutely ideal whole-food biscuit, as are many crispbreads. There are also the polystyrene-lookalike rice cakes, which are comprised of pieces of puffed rice stuck together. They are actually rather tasty, but the texture is one that some people love and others do not care for at all. They are especially useful if you suspect you may have a wheat or gluten allergy, and can be eaten with pâtés, spreads and jams.

By distinct contrast, most sweet biscuits are full of sugar and fat. You are far better off making your own, although you may find you have to be quite creative in order to bake good whole-food vegan biscuits. In general terms, the best ones to go for are oat, fruit and nut-based biscuits of the flapjack type, or wholemeal digestives. It is also possible to use stewed fruit purées and chopped nuts to make moister, more interesting and more delicious biscuits, if you feel so inclined.

DRIED FRUITS

Dried fruits have been mentioned in the context of lovely things to have at breakfast time alongside your muesli, such as dried apricots, figs and prunes. Of course, there are also dried peaches, pears, dates, raisins and sultanas. The undisputed king of the raisins is the very large lexia raisin, which is absolutely delicious. Lexia raisins can also be soaked and eaten as a fruit compote, either on their own or mixed with other dried or fresh fruits.

Dried bananas, mangoes and pineapples are also available but, to my taste, these are so far from the originals that I cannot really get too excited about them. Some people love them, though, either on their own as an alternative to sweets, or mixed in muesli and desserts.

The issue with dried fruits is the fact that, being so sticky and sweet, they are extremely susceptible to attack by moulds and bacteria in transit. As a result, many of them are covered in sulphur, oils, insecticides and pesticides. Again, it is best to go organic if possible. You will tend to find that really organic dried fruit is dried more than treated fruit, so that it is less sticky and therefore less vulnerable to attack. This will mean it is less succulent to eat raw, but will probably reconstitute just as well if left to soak. A good example of this is the hunza apricot already described, which, although sold in a rather tough, dry, nut-like state, will soften after the two-day soaking process described (*see page 36*) into the most succulent, delicious dessert imaginable.

It is rather nice to make your own jams and spreads by puréeing stewed dried fruits. As mentioned before, these can form delicious bases or toppings for pies, tarts and desserts, especially if cooked with a touch of ginger, bay, cardamom, cinnamon or other spices of your choice.

SPICES AND FLAVOURINGS

There are far too many herbs and spices to discuss them individually, but again the best advice here is to try if you can to grow some herbs of your own, such as basil, coriander, mint and chives in the summer, and rosemary, sage and thyme all the year round.

Two other absolute cornerstones of most vegetarian cookery are garlic and root ginger. It is even possible to find or make ginger juice, which is like a ginger essence that can be added to recipes. You can also grow or buy horseradish root, which has a very lively flavour grated into vegetables or sauces.

For most people, the main problem is what to do about replacing salt. Luckily, there is a range of possible alternatives. Soy sauce, shoyu and tamari are liquid and can be sprinkled over most dishes to add a salty flavour. Miso is a brown paste which needs to be mixed with water and then stirred into dishes to flavour them. It can also be used to make a soup or a savoury drink. These substances are still quite high in salt, but of course have other nutrients – particularly minerals – which make using them much better than using pure salt. Miso is often mixed with rice or barley and, coming primarily from the soya bean, is a rich source of protein and other valuable nutrients.

Another helpful source of flavouring can be found in yeast extracts such as *Vecon*. These take the place of stock cubes, though again, are rather high in salt so should be used judiciously. A teaspoon of *Vecon* with some boiling water can form a very pleasant savoury alternative to a cup of tea on a cold night! This can also be achieved with half a teaspoon of vegetable bouillon powder (such as *Marigold*) and further enhanced with some sliced root ginger, which is a great immune stimulant.

The vinegar family is a rich source of flavouring. Of course, in Britain we are most familiar with harsh malt vinegars, but there are the much softer, more delicate cider and tarragon vinegars, and the absolutely delicious balsamic vinegar which is matured in oak caskets in Italy. This makes it much sweeter and more delicately flavoured than most vinegars, and absolutely ideal for most dressings and recipes requiring vinegar. For an interesting change it is also possible to get fruit vinegars, such as raspberry vinegar; this, with a little walnut oil, can make a wonderful salad dressing.

While on the subject of salad dressings, I have mentioned already that it is advisable not to use too much oil. As a substitute, try fresh organic or silken tofu mixed with some onion, vinegar, mustard and a herb of your choice.

Mustards and mustard seeds are a very good source of flavour and can be used in all sorts of recipes. Particularly good are the wholegrain mustards, or the fine French Dijon mustard, which can give a nicely piquant edge to a sauce.

Another idea is to use pre-made curry sauces, masalas, chutneys and pickles in your recipes. These can sometimes add a sweet/sour dimension to food, which can make it very interesting. Pre-made curry sauces, particularly the authentic Indian ones found in Indian shops, can instantly transform a vegetable stew into a vegetable curry.

For the adventurous there is also the possibility of using seaweeds to flavour your cooking. These can be added to vegetables, rice or grains, with delicious results. The most commonly found seaweeds in health-food shops are nori, combu, arame, wakame and hijiki. There is no way to describe the flavour of these seaweeds. Very broadly speaking, the best results I have achieved are by toasting the seaweeds lightly and then crumbling and sprinkling them over rice, grains, bakes or casseroles.

If you find you are absolutely unable to give up salt, a way of cutting down greatly is to make *gomasio*. For this you grind toasted sesame seeds (that is, sesame seeds which have been roasted on a baking tray in a hot oven or tossed in a frying pan until they are deep brown) with a little sea salt (in a ratio of about 10 parts sesame seeds to

1 part sea salt). This is absolutely delicious and will convey a great deal of flavour without too high a salt content.

The other bit of good news is that it is still possible to include a little home-made mayonnaise in your diet. One egg yolk will hold about a quarter of a pint of olive oil beaten in drop by drop; to this you can add some balsamic vinegar or just lemon juice and, if you wish, some garlic. A small amount of this dropped into a bowl of tomato soup will enrich it beyond belief, adding tremendous texture and flavour, or of course it can be eaten with salads or on top of baked potatoes.

Another staple for most vegetarian cooks is the tomato in its many forms. Perhaps most useful is tomato purée, which can be used to add flavour to many recipes. Another luxurious member of this family is the fashionable sun-dried tomato, which is highly flavoured and can be used to bring all sorts of recipes alive. The same goes for the olive family. It is now possible to get all manner of good olives in Britain, but I think my favourite for flavour is the kalamata olive, which is firm, juicy and extremely tasty. Real lovers of olives will adore olive pâté, which is available in good health-food stores and delicatessens and can be used in all sorts of ways to enrich food; it can also be eaten as it is on a cracker or with raw vegetables as a snack. It is now also possible to get basil purée, which means that you can have the wonderful fresh basil taste even in the dead of winter.

Mushrooms are, of course, a subject in their own right. Many books have been written on mushroom cookery alone. I mention mushrooms here because often a very small amount can flavour an entire risotto or pasta dish. Special mushrooms include the French cepes, pleurotes or oyster mushrooms, bolets and the Chinese shiitake mushroom. Many of these are available dried; they reconstitute well when soaked and can then be sliced for use in stir-fries and other dishes where their flavour goes a very long way.

CHEESE

'Vegetarian cheese' is a bit of a misnomer. What this usually means is that it is ordinary cheese made as usual from dairy produce, but without rennet in it. The reason for this is that vegetarians who do not eat meat on ethical grounds will not tolerate rennet, as it is extracted from the calf's stomach. It is an enzyme which helps convert the milk drunk by the calf into a more solid cheese-like form of protein for digestive purposes. This makes it very useful for initiating the process of turning milk into cheese commercially. The only real vegetarian, or should I say vegan, cheese is again made from soya – surprise, surprise! However, this is not really much like ordinary cheese and its use is somewhat analogous to using TVP 'mince' and 'steak'. In general, it is far better to get used to genuine alternatives, such as hummus and vegetable pâtés, rather than a pale imitation of the real thing!

Cheeses made from sheep's and goat's milk are more likely to be organic than those made from cow's milk, and goat's-milk cheese has the lowest fat content of all three. However, they are still best avoided if you are to keep your diet low in animal fats and protein. Some cheese addicts attain high cheese flavour with low cheese intake by using a small grating of Parmesan on their bakes, rather than any other type of cheese.

SNACKS AND SWEETS

Nuts are the most obvious whole-food snacks, but they should be eaten unsalted and without dry-roasted additive coatings! There is also a large and ever-growing range of whole-food crisps and tortilla chips. However, it is worth checking the list of ingredients to make sure they do not contain chemical additives, colourings and flavourings. Poppadums also make a nice snack and can be used for dips. Rice crackers, too, can be used for this purpose, but again look at the list of ingredients for the good ones.

Most whole-food sweets are based around nuts, dried fruit and seeds. Good examples are simply mixed fresh fruits and nuts, or nut bars, sesame snacks, dried fruit bars or halva, which is made from crushed sesame seeds and honey. There is, of course, also liquorice and liquorice sticks, which some people love to chew. It is advisable to get your children going on these kinds of sweets if at all possible before they acquire too great a taste for the extremely sugary sweets which are commonly available.

It is also possible to get or make pure fruit juice ice-lollies, which again are far better than the synthetically-flavoured and highly sweetened ones. They are also far superior to dairy ice cream, which is packed full of animal fats and additives.

BABY FOODS

It is surprisingly easy to find whole-food, vegetarian baby foods. You will be pleased to hear that there are now many ranges of organic baby foods available in the UK (the first well-recognized brand name was *Organix*). Good-quality baby milks such as *Wysoy* are made from enriched soya milk. Many of the foods described already in the 'Breakfast Cereals' and 'Beans' sections will make very good purées for babies starting on solids, if mixed with vegetables or fruit purées and juices as appropriate. Soya yoghurts and desserts are also acceptable to most babies. The notion that babies love sugary things is inspired by our adult viewpoint: most babies will lap up healthy alternatives, and the whole-food habit will stick if started early enough.

There is an opinion that too much soya milk may not be good for babies because it contains plant oestrogens. These can, theoretically, block the child's own oestrogen activity, which is related to sexual development. However, there is no evidence whatsoever that any child reared on soya milk has suffered ill-effects of this kind.

FRUITS AND VEGETABLES

There are far too many fruits and vegetables even to begin to enumerate them here. The key, as mentioned before, is to go with what is available locally and in season, with as great an emphasis as possible on buying food that's fresh and organic. Once you become confident with a few basic recipes, branch out and begin learning to bake and stuff vegetables such as marrows, aubergines and peppers. When you get more ambitious, try looking around Chinese and Indian supermarkets, where you will find more exciting challenges and flavours.

Planning and Shopping

Now you have had a glimpse of the enormous variety open to you, perhaps you are prepared to commit yourself to making the changeover straightaway. Perhaps, on the other hand, you feel that you are going to have to make the change gradually, in stages.

I will now describe a step-by-step process to help you decide exactly how far you want to go, how soon, and what help you will need. Just because you may not be able to take on board all the changes immediately does not invalidate those you are ready to make.

STEP ONE – DECISION TIME

The first step is for you to decide how far you are going to take it, and so I advise you to check down the following list and answer these questions for yourself:

1   Am I going to stop eating meat altogether?
2   Am I going to stop eating chicken and game?
3   Am I going to stop eating fish and shellfish?

4 Am I going to stop consuming milk?

5 Am I going to stop consuming butter?

6 Am I going to stop consuming dairy yoghurt?

7 Am I going to stop eating cheese?

8 Am I going to stop eating cream?

9 Am I going to stop drinking coffee?

10 Am I going to stop drinking tea?

11 Am I going to stop using salt?

12 Am I going to stop using sugar?

13 Am I going to stop eating refined and processed foods?

14 Am I committed to decreasing my protein and fat intake?

15 Am I committed to raising my intake of fruit, vegetables, cereals and pulses?

16 Am I committed to drinking fresh spring or bottled water daily?

STEP TWO – THE MASTER PLAN

I now suggest that you write your decisions out for yourself as a positive plan: in other words, for example in response to question 1 – 'I intend to stop eating red meat'; question 2 – 'I intend to stop eating chicken'; and so on down the list. This will really clarify and affirm your intention, and can be modified every few months as the change becomes easier and your intention becomes stronger. It may even help you to read your intention to yourself every few days, to strengthen your resolve.

STEP THREE – SUPPORT

The next step is to decide how much support you are going to need. First of all, it would help to show your 'positive plan' of statements to your family or a partner or friend, and see if they are prepared to change with you. If not, explain to them how best they can support you and also how they can avoid sabotaging you. If you cook together, perhaps suggest they wait to cook their food until after you have cooked yours, or that they avoid buying things which are most likely to tempt you until you are well established in your new way of eating. Perhaps they could join you temporarily while you get started, or could take on learning one or two recipes so that you can have a couple of nights per week off from having to prepare your own meals. Perhaps you can find somebody else – a friend, colleague or someone you have met at a support group if you are ill – who will embark upon the new way of eating with you.

The next question is whether you feel you are going to need a counsellor, nutritional therapist or doctor to see you regularly through this period of transition, especially if you think you may be compulsive about food, tend to use food as a sedative, or if you have a medical or treatment consideration which may affect the process. If you need help or advice in finding a suitable counsellor, nutritional therapist or holistic doctor, please do not hesitate to contact Health Creation's helpline (0117 949 3363), or visit our website at HealthCreation.co.uk.

STEP FOUR – THE GAME PLAN

The next thing to do is decide how you are going to tackle this. Many people find that it is easiest to change one meal at a time, perhaps starting with breakfast and then going on to lunch and finally dinner. This may not suit you and you may instead choose to make the change in one go; again, make your intentions clear to those around you. It is also easier to start by adding healthy foods to your diet before you take away the unhealthy ones. For example, you could start by making sure you eat fruit several times a day, and have vegetables and a salad as part of your two main meals. You could then go 'whole food' – cutting out refined foods then gradually introducing more cereals, grains and pulses, and finally dropping meat, dairy produce, salt and sugar.

STEP FIVE – HALFWAY THERE ALREADY!

The next step is to identify as far as possible which foods, dishes and recipes you already know and like, and which fit into your master plan. Do not forget, for example, that simple things such as baked beans on toast, lentil soup, baked potatoes or porridge with honey fall into this category, as do most salads, fruit salads and many pasta dishes.

You may be quite surprised at how many things you already eat are vegan, and how many of your usual recipes can easily be 'converted' with the use of meat substitutes. For example, it is possible to make a pasta bolognese or a shepherd's pie with TVP mince. It is also possible in the early days to have veggie burgers with brown rolls, relish and salad, so changing over to a healthier way of eating may not be quite as gruesome as you think!

STEP SIX – MEAL PLANNING

I have already described an ideal whole-food breakfast comprised of muesli, cereals or porridge; stewed fruit or fresh fruit (possibly in a fruit salad) with soya yoghurt; whole-wheat toast or fruit breads with margarine and low-sugar jams and honey, nut or seed spreads; accompanied by fruit juice or herb teas. Occasionally, you may wish to have a cooked breakfast, with perhaps vegetarian sausages, mushrooms, grilled tomatoes and maybe an egg.

You will have to decide for yourself which will be your main meal of the day. As stated earlier, it is better to have the main meal at midday, but this may not be possible in the context of your working life. If this is the case, then the ideal lunch to aim for may well be a vegetable lentil or bean soup accompanied by a salad made from salad vegetables, beans or rice. A possible alternative would be well-thought-out and delicious sandwiches, which could contain vegetarian pâté or hummus with salad, olives or avocados. You may prefer a vegetable pie or pasty, or even a light pasta dish with salad. This can be followed with fresh fruit or freshly made fruit juice, or a soya dessert.

For your main meal you have many choices, starting with simple stir-fried vegetable dishes with rice or other grains, bean or lentil stews or casseroles, pasta dishes (including vegetarian lasagne), shepherd's pie, vegetarian curries or chilli, vegetable bakes or crumbles, pies, nut roasts, risottos and perhaps the occasional grilled fish dish with vegetables. Of course, there are also all the convenience foods like non-meat pies, vegetarian sausages and so on.

You can probably cover yourself quite well for breakfast and lunches by shopping regularly for cereals, dried fruits, fruit spreads and basic vegetables from which to make soups, and a good variety of lunchtime salads. It is also possible now to buy very good 'home-made' vegetable soups in most supermarkets – for example the *Covent Garden* range of soups. Choose soups such as lentil, bean or winter vegetable, however, which do not contain large amounts of cream and butter! To get yourself going for main meals it may then be advisable to write down a list of at least seven main meal dishes that you either know already or can learn to prepare before you make the change altogether. At the point at which you have mastered seven main meal recipes, you have probably acquired the minimum basic skills to make the change.

You may like to check which foods contain certain vitamins and minerals so that you can put extra thought into the planning of your meals. With this in mind, here is a table that should help:

A (Retinol & Beta Carotene)	Protects against infections, antioxidant & immune system booster, protects against many forms of cancer	carrots, watercress, cabbage, squash, sweet potato, melon, pumpkin, tomato, broccoli, apricots, papayas
B (Ergocalciferol)	Helps maintain strong and healthy bones by retaining calcium	herring, mackerel, salmon, other fish, eggs
E (D-alpha tocopheral)	Antioxidant, protecting cells from damage, including cancer; helps body use oxygen, preventing blood clots, improves wound healing, good for the skin	unrefined vegetable oils, seeds, nuts, beans, peas, wheat germ, whole grains, fatty fish, tuna, mackerel, salmon, sweet potato
K (Phylloquinine)	Controls blood clotting	cauliflower, Brussels sprouts, lettuce, cabbage, beans, broccoli, peas, watercress, asparagus, potato, tomatoes
C (Ascorbic acid)	Strengthens the immune system, fights infections, makes collagen (keeping bones, skin and joints firm and strong), antioxidant (detoxifying pollutants and protecting against cancer and heart disease), helps make anti-stress hormones and turn food into energy	sweet peppers, watercress, cabbage, broccoli, cauliflower, strawberries, lemons, peas, melons, oranges, grapefruit, limes, tomatoes
B1 (Thiamine)	Essential for energy production, brain function and digestion, helps the body make use of protein	watercress, squash, courgettes, asparagus, mushrooms, peas, lettuce, sweet peppers, cauliflower, cabbage, tomatoes, Brussels sprouts, beans
B3 (Niacin)	Helps balance blood sugar and lower cholesterol levels, also involved in inflammation and digestion	mushrooms, tuna, salmon, asparagus, cabbage, mackerel, tomatoes, squash, courgettes, cauliflower and unrefined cereals
B6 (Pyrodixine)	Essential for protein digestion and utilization, brain function, hormone production; natural antidepressant and diuretic, helps control allergic reaction	watercress, cauliflower, cabbage, peppers, bananas, squash, broccoli, asparagus, lentils, Brussels sprouts, onions, seeds and nuts
B12 (Cyanocobalamin)	Needed for using protein, helps blood carry oxygen, essential for nerves, detoxifies tobacco smoke and other toxins	fish, oysters, sardines, tuna, eggs, shrimps

STEP SEVEN – THE SHOPPING LIST

You will find life a great deal easier if you make yourself a basic shopping list which you stick to your kitchen wall and which you can check against each time you make your shopping list. When we have been cooking one way for a long time we have a mental checklist from which we make our shopping list, and of course this will now be different. You may also want to make yourself a 'don't buy' list, sticking it next to the other list to reinforce your good intentions. Although there is an increasing amount of vegan foods available from major supermarkets, I would still suggest you take time to go and visit the best health-food shops you can find in your area. If you have never been to one of these shops before, it will probably make quite an impact as you become aware of the large selection of foods available to you. This will contrast sharply with the experience of going around a supermarket seeking out the healthy food from among hundreds of items which do not fit into a healthy eating plan.

The following can be used as a 'master list' to check against each week:

Organic wholemeal bread

Fruit bread

Savoury biscuits, crispbread, rice cakes or oat cakes

Whole-food digestive biscuits

Whole-food cake

Soya milk

Soya yoghurt

Soya dessert (e.g. *Provamel*)

Organic eggs

Margarine (*Granose* or *Vitaquel*)

Oil (olive, peanut, speciality nut oils)

Tea – *Luaka*, decaffeinated Earl Grey, herbal, fruit

Barleycup, Yannoh, Bambu

Mineral water

Fruit juice

Fruit spread (sugar-free)

Marmalade (sugar-free)

Honey

Tahini

Peanut butter

Hummus

Vegetable pâté or spreads (such as *Tartex*)

Whole flours

Brown rice

Lentils

Beans

Cereals

Porridge oats (ordinary or jumbo)

Muesli (unsweetened natural muesli from health-food shops)

Nuts

Seeds

Dried fruits

Pasta (dried or freshly prepared)

Noodles

Pasta sauces

Pickles (in moderation)

Mustard

Mayonnaise

Vinegar (including balsamic, fruit or cider vinegar)

Chilli sauce

Soy sauce

Chinese sauces (such as yellow bean paste, black bean paste)

Miso

Marigold low-salt bouillon powder

Black peppercorns

Herbs and spices

Garlic and ginger

Tomato purée

Chestnut purée

Coconut cream

Tinned tomatoes

Tinned red kidney beans or other pulses

Tinned sweetcorn

Vegetables – roots, greens

Salad

Fruit

Bean curd

Quorn – mince, chunks or 'sausage meat'

TVP sausages/bacon

TVP mince, chunks or 'sausage meat'

Fish

Pre-made soups

Pre-made pies, pasties and bakes

Ideal Meals

I have mentioned again and again that we need to get away from the Western idea of basing our meals around a big hunk of protein. So what is the ideal meal?

Try thinking about the way the Chinese and Indians eat. Very small amounts of protein are cooked in sauces and then served with large amounts of rice, breads and vegetables. The idea is really to make sure that the major input in each meal is a mixture of carbohydrate and vegetables, or fruit. Roughly speaking, the carbohydrate element should form around 40 per cent of each meal, the vegetables around 40 per cent, protein around 10–15 per cent, and fat around 5 per cent. For example, some beans cooked in a tomato or vegetable sauce served on a bed of rice with a large side salad would be ideal. Alternatively, some stir-fried vegetables served with brown rice and braised tofu or stir-fried Quorn would be good. Pilau rice with nuts added to it, accompanied by a vegetable curry and dahl, also makes for an extremely well-balanced meal; or perhaps some soup and salad with hummus and brown bread.

You will soon discover that by eating this way you will never feel bloated or nauseated after a meal, and that you will not experience peaks and troughs of energy in the same way as you do on refined foods. The energy you receive from your food will be of good quality and enduring as the food is digested over a period of hours. Gradually, you will feel stronger, healthier and far more alert.

Timing of meals

Try very hard to get into the habit of eating three meals a day, and if possible have your main meal around midday. Make time for your meals so that you can eat slowly and enjoy your food, and, particularly, leave adequate time for digestion after your meal. Try not to eat your evening meal much later than 7 p.m. so that you can allow time for digestion before you go to bed.

RAPID FOOD PREPARATION

The reason many people give for finding it difficult to become vegan or vegetarian is the time taken to prepare meals. I can assure you that once you are in the habit of eating in this way, preparing meals will take you no longer than usual. However, there are tips which will help you.

First, it is very useful to keep some pre-cooked beans and rice in the fridge. When you cook either rice or beans, cook more than you need and coat the remainder with a little bit of olive oil. You can then use either the rice or beans to make a very quick salad, simply adding chopped apples, sweetcorn, red or green peppers, onions, etc. to the rice, or a little onion, garlic, parsley and tomato to the beans. With the addition of an oil and vinegar vinaigrette, you have a wonderful instant meal.

It is also possible to reheat the rice or beans for use in stews (beans) or fried-rice dishes. Simply make a sauce with onions, tomatoes, garlic, tomato purée and herbs, and add in the beans. In this way you can have a main course meal in the time it takes to cook your rice. Of course, tinned beans can be used in this way, too, as a convenience food. It is also possible to freeze rice and beans for reuse in these ways, or to make large quantities of bean stews, vegetable curries and pasta sauces and keep them in the freezer.

I must stress again, however, that the freezer should not be viewed as anything other than a long-term fridge, as the food quality will deteriorate. Aim to eat frozen food within three weeks of freezing it. If you can possibly make food fresh, it is by far the better course.

A food processor will vastly reduce the time involved in making vegetable salads, and if you keep a jar of vinaigrette in the fridge you can have a meal prepared in minutes. It is also possible to buy salad ready prepared from major supermarkets, although this is a rather expensive way of buying your salad.

Pasta meals can be ready within 10 to 15 minutes if you use a pre-made tomato sauce, for example. While the pasta is boiling you can make a salad, get the dressing out of the fridge and sprinkle some over it. It is also a good idea to make a big pot of soup once or twice a week. *Vecon* or *Marigold Bouillon* powder, which are vegetable stocks, can be used for extra flavouring. Quite a good tip is to purée half of the pot of soup in a food processor or blender and return this half to the pot, leaving the remaining thin cooking liquid as it is and the other vegetable pieces whole. This will give you a soup with a nice creamy texture and some bits of whole vegetable for texture. If you purée the entire contents of the pot, the soup sometimes becomes far too thick and heavy.

The classic easy soups to master are lentil (made with red lentils, onions and tomatoes), leek and potato (vichyssoise) and onion. These three soups are very simple and absolutely delicious. If you take the time to prepare a lot of any one soup, you can have two or three meals stored in the refrigerator or freezer and ready to be reheated in minutes – and, of course, soups and stews improve if left to stand overnight.

Snack attacks

The second thing which floors many people's attempts to become vegetarian is the 'snack attack'. The things people are used to reaching for are cheese and crackers, sweet biscuits, cakes, crisps, salami, meat pâtés and chocolate. Part of this whole syndrome is the fact, as previously explained, that eating the wrong sort of food causes blood-sugar levels to swing between very high and very low, producing the tendency to want to snack or binge between meals. In this way we can easily end up taking in over twice as many calories as we need every day, and putting on far too much weight in the process, not to mention leaving ourselves feeling permanently exhausted.

However, we are never going to get away entirely from the need for snacks, and so it is better to be prepared with tempting, instantly available whole-food goodies, than to relapse into old habits.

The ideal foods for this are crispbreads and oatcakes with hummus, vegetable pâté, yeast pâtés (for example *Tartex*), olive pâté and basil pâté. Having a good supply of first-class olives can also do the trick, or alternatively some delicious nuts or seeds. Ideally, some pistachios, pine kernels, peanuts, cashews or macadamia nuts would be wonderful; tamari-toasted sunflower seeds are excellent too. Some people prefer a mixture of dried fruits and nuts, such as peanuts with raisins and sultanas. Dried fruit itself is excellent for snacking: the best candidates are dried figs, peaches and apricots.

There are many whole-food crisps or tortilla chips made purely from wheat and water, but do check you are not buying products full of additives and salt. The other solution is to make crudités out of raw vegetables such as sweet peppers, celery or carrots, using these to dip into something like hummus or a vegetable purée. The most important thing here is to think ahead and be prepared, so that you always have something in the fridge or cupboard when a snack attack strikes!

FAMILY TIPS

If you live with your family, the ages of your family members will make an enormous difference to their willingness to accept the shift towards vegan food. Nowadays, many teenagers are becoming vegetarians of their own accord, due to the extensive education in schools and on television about environmental issues. On the other hand, there are many teenagers who are extremely clear about their desire to eat meat, not to change their eating habits, and particularly not to do anything you (their parents) are doing. Usually, if they are old enough to be this clear, they are probably old enough to have some input into their own cooking, and I strongly recommend that you let go somewhat of your role of provider and allow them to cook their own meals. Very young children, for their part, are usually quite amenable to things such as bean and vegetable purées and soya yoghurts and desserts. Somewhere in between these extremes, perhaps between the ages of 5 and 13, is the difficult patch. These children are usually extremely rigid in their eating patterns and highly influenced by peer pressure. With this group, the key is keeping everything looking and feeling as 'normal' as usual, and this is where things like TVP sausages, mince, steak chunks and vegetarian meat pies are worth their weight in gold.

It is always advisable to make changes as slowly and imperceptibly as possible, and to resist the urge to lecture your children about what's good for them – this will inevitably lead to stubborn resistance to all your efforts! Fortunately, the media nowadays is more and more onto the healthy eating tack. School catering, however, is often still in the dark ages; it may be worthwhile trying to get involved with influencing the meal policy in your children's school by doing a little lobbying via the school's parent-teacher group or board of governors. If your child takes a packed lunch to school, so much the better.

VARIETY AND SEASON

While you will be ready to start your vegan lifestyle once you have mastered seven main dish recipes, your aim should be to go on experimenting and diversifying your range of meals. It is very important, both nutritionally and for your own sense of creativity, to continue to explore and try new things, and eating a good range of foods will ensure you get a nutritionally balanced diet. It is also wise to change your eating patterns with the seasons and eat what is fresh at the different times of year. Fresh foods contain by far the most nutrients and vitality, and their flavour will also be best. The other distinct advantages about buying foods in season are that of course they will be far cheaper and you will not get bored.

Gradually, as you become more adventurous about experimenting with colours and flavours and new techniques, herbs, spices and foods from different cultures, you will realize that cooking in this way is infinitely exciting and satisfying, enabling you to feel happier and healthier than ever before, and really comfortable in your body.

Stress and 'Failure'

The holistic approach to cancer prevention revolves first and foremost around reducing stress and increasing our happiness, fulfilment and pleasure.

It is very easy to see how changing the way we eat and giving up a lot of our favourite things can appear to be completely opposed to this underlying principle. There is also the definite risk that those of you who are very frightened by the thought of cancer can cling on to this dietary advice, becoming rigid and obsessive and stressing yourselves terribly if you lapse or are unable to maintain this healthy way of eating. It is extremely important to remember that the way we eat is only one part of the picture, and that the most important thing of all is that we are gentle with ourselves. If you are finding it hard to adapt to healthy eating, it may mean that you are pushing yourself too fast, and perhaps don't yet have sufficient support or information to make a sudden, big change to your diet and eating habits. There may be an emotional or stress-related factor that perhaps needs attention first. Remember that it can be better to start with small changes than to try to completely transform your eating habits overnight and fail.

However, as with all other areas of life, having the fundamental intention to move towards healthy eating patterns is the real foundation stone for the process. This will, for some, take weeks; for others it may take years. A wise friend of mine was asked about the process of creating intention: 'How can 10 minutes a day of visualizing the way I want things to be possibly influence the other rubbish I am thinking the other 23 hours and 50 minutes?' To this he replied, 'If a dog catches the whiff of something good on the wind and his nose turns towards where the good smell is coming from, then all the rest of him has to follow.' This is also true of good intentions. If you re-read your new diet decisions every few weeks and reaffirm your choices to yourself, I assure you the changes will gradually take place.

The other thing to remember with nutrition is that it is what you eat the majority of the time that will make the difference, so the occasional lapse in your diet does not mean you have failed. What you will find interesting, in fact, is that if you decide to have steak and chips followed by gateau and double cream one night after you have been following the whole-foods diet for a while, it will be very clear what this does to your body as it attempts to cope once more with the physiological stress of digesting large amounts of protein, fat and sugar! So the odd binge can actually have a very helpful effect in showing you the benefits of your new way of eating.

Seriously, though, be kind to yourself and do not 'beat yourself up' if you stray from the path for a few days. Once you realize this has happened, perhaps get help or more support, maybe see a nutritional therapist again to get more encouragement, or repeat the process of making a master plan which is more realistic and simpler for you to stick with. By continuing to repeat this process every two to three months, you will ultimately come out with the perfect diet for your individual needs.

Ideas for a Week's Menu – by Jane Sen

Once you are gaining in confidence, you may like to try creating for yourself a week's menu from the following ideas. All these recipes can be found in Chapter 5:

BREAKFAST IDEAS

1 Fresh fruit and/or vegetable juice
   Hot porridge made with soya milk and oats or brown rice (other grains are good, too: try cracked wheat or millet) served with dried fruits (prunes, apricots, figs, dates, raisins, apples, pears) soaked overnight in apple juice or water with or without some chopped mixed nuts

2 Fresh fruit and/or vegetable juice
   Granola-style cereal with soya milk and a sliced banana or two, or some fresh figs
   Slice of wholemeal bread, spread with *Vitam R* or *Vecon* and piled with thick sliced fresh tomato and a drizzle of olive oil, then popped under a hot grill for 5 minutes

3 Fruit salad of four or five mixed fresh fruits sprinkled with nuts (toasted coconut is lovely)

Toast or rice cakes with low-salt spreads, bean pâté or nut butter

4 Fresh fruit and/or vegetable juice

Baked beans on wholemeal toast

Crispbread with unsweetened fruit spreads or honey

Fresh pear or apple

5 Soya dessert (e.g. *Provamel*) served with fresh fruit sauce (e.g. bananas, peaches, strawberries, apricots, raspberries, apples, pears, whizzed together in the blender or food processor), sprinkled with a little Granola-style cereal or toasted nuts and seeds

Toasted muffins or fruit bread with soya margarine and unsweetened fruit spread

6 Fresh fruit and/or vegetable juice

Compote of dried fruits (apricots, dates, figs, pineapple, mango, prunes, berries, apples, raisins), either soaked overnight in apple juice or water, or cooked very gently until soft, eaten warm or cold. Serve with oat or rice milk, or, for extra luxury, nut cream and/or pancakes

7 Fresh fruit and/or vegetable juice

Organic cornflakes or cereal with soya milk

Toasted wholemeal bread topped with slices of tofu, drizzled with tamari or tahini and popped under a hot grill with a sliced tomato to brown

Fresh fruits

8 Fresh fruit and/or vegetable juice, muesli with hot or cold soya milk (try soaking the muesli in the milk overnight to make it extra creamy and digestible)

Toast or rice cakes with a mashed banana sprinkled with toasted sesame, poppy or sunflower seeds

Main meals

1 Creamy Leek and Mushroom Croustade

Ginger and Sesame Carrots

Lightly cooked green vegetable

Tomato and cucumber salad with Parsley Vinaigrette

Fresh pears with almond 'cream' or soya dessert

2 Stir-fry of Asparagus and Brazil Nuts

Brown rice or noodles, with grated raw carrots and chopped spring onions stirred in before serving

Shredded Chinese leaf, celery and bean sprouts with Orange and Sesame Dressing

Compote of dried apricots (just cover with apple juice and simmer gently until soft), served with Orange Spice Cream

3 Moroccan-style Braised Vegetables and Butter Beans

Steamed couscous or bulgar

Mixed green leaf salad with garlic vinaigrette

Fresh strawberries and peaches, or apples and oranges served with banana 'cream'

4 Malay-spiced Tofu

Braised Sweet and Sour Carrots

Rice or noodles with an equal volume of fine shredded watercress stirred in just before serving

Spinach and Sunflower Seed Salad

Poached pears with fresh strawberry or raspberry coulis

5 Galette of Parsnips and Cashew Nuts

Creamed fennel or potatoes

Lightly cooked green vegetables

Perfectly Pink Salad

Fresh fruit salad (made up of at least four different fruits)

6 Tagliatelle with 'Creamy' Mushroom Sauce

Grilled vegetables (aubergines, onions, tomatoes, courgettes, etc.) in Mustard Sauce

Mixed green leaf and cucumber salad with fresh tomato dressing

Stuffed Baked Apples with Blackberry Sauce

7   Potato and mushroom curry
    Spiced lentils of your choice
    Rice or quinoa with shredded, steamed or raw spinach
    Chopped tomatoes, cucumber and pink onions in 'creamy' mint dressing
    Juicy fresh pineapple

8   Braised Squash with Green Lentils
    Aromatic Glazed Turnips
    Warm Cauliflower Salad
    Fine shredded red and white cabbage salad
    Italian Almond Pudding

LIGHT MEALS

1   Fresh Corn Chowder
    Hot granary bread
    Warm Red Cabbage Salad with Watercress and Toasted Pecans
    Two pieces of your favourite fruit

2   Poppy Seed and Sour 'Cream' Pasta
    Tomato, onion and olive salad with tiny leaf cress
    Fresh melon

3   Parsnip 'Dabs' with sweet red pepper sauce
    Steamed or lightly cooked broccoli
    Indonesian Sprout and Nut Salad
    Fresh pineapple and oranges

4   Grilled Aubergines with Salsa Verde
    Middle Eastern Rice Salad
    Fresh peaches, plums or apricots

5 Courgette and Potato Rosti
   Broccoli, Macadamia and Garlic Salad
   Fresh tomatoes
   Soya dessert

6 Quinoa pilaf
   Good All Round Tomato Sauce
   Mixed green leaf salad
   'Creamy' avocado dressing
   Fresh grapes

7 Wholemeal bread or pitta bread stuffed with hummus, Tunisian-style carrot salad
   and shredded lettuce
   Slice of banana and hazelnut cake

8 'Creamy' Cauliflower Soup
   Spicy Oven 'Fries'
   Warm Red Cabbage Salad with Watercress and Toasted Pecans
   Dried apricots, dates and figs

CHAPTER 4

Food as Therapy

The relationship between food and health can be seen along a spectrum, with healthy eating (which is relevant to everyone) at one end of the spectrum, and food used as medicine or therapy at the other.

When food is used as therapy, very specific, usually very rigid dietary regimes are advised with a view to detoxifying the body, dramatically raising one's energy levels, correcting energetic imbalances, rectifying nutritional imbalances by replacing deficient vitamins, minerals or other nutrients, or using a food, vitamin, mineral or nutrient as a medicine in its own right.

The other type of food therapy is the category of exclusion diets, where rather than adding foods to a diet, items are withdrawn in order to see whether they are having an irritant or allergic effect on an individual's system.

Food is probably the oldest form of medicine that we have. Human beings from every single culture have realized the connections between what we eat, how we feel, whether we get sick and how we can be helped. This makes it all the more extraordinary that the role of nutritional medicine seems to have been virtually ignored by modern Western medicine.

The bottom line is that, as with any high-performance machine, the performance of the body is directly affected by the fuel we put into it. Our bodies tell us in a variety of ways when the foods we are eating are not meeting our nutritional requirements, through the state of our skin, hair and nails, our energy levels, our gut's performance, and symptoms such as nausea, irritability, irritable bowel, palpitations, allergic reactions and in many other ways.

There are two main problems – one is that very often those with a strong will or a determined or perhaps stoical spirit will chronically override signals from the body that all is not well. This, coupled with a great deal of ignorance among the medical profession as to the symptoms of nutritional imbalance and poor diet, and a tendency to treat these problems with drugs and procedures which often only make the situation worse, can often lead to the root of these problems going undiscovered, in some cases for a whole lifetime!

Apart from nutritional imbalance and deficiency, there is also the increasing problem of allergies, as foods become more complex, more processed and more changed by cooking and preservation processes. When this problem combines with the absorption of many other toxic chemicals from our environment as well as extreme stress and the long-term compromising of the workings of the digestive system, all sorts of problems and pathologies develop, including many of the auto-immune diseases, allergic conditions, cancer and arterial disease.

Nutritional Therapy

A good, well-qualified nutritional therapist is trained to understand the signs and signals the body is giving us, and to tell you exactly where the deficiencies are in your diet, whether or not you are experiencing allergic symptoms, digestive problems or even infection with *Candida Albicans* (yeast) in the gut as a result of the way you are eating. He or she will also be able to give you the necessary support and information to alter your diet so that you can bring your system back into balance. This approach can be backed up by analyses of blood, sweat and hair samples, by firms such as Biolab (9 Weymouth Street, London W1W 6DB), to measure the levels of minerals and vitamins in your system. In this way your progress can be monitored regularly. Blood and sweat analyses will give you a very up-to-the-minute picture of how your body is coping, whereas analysis of hair samples will give you a slightly more historical picture of what has or has not been laid down over the preceding weeks.

It is also possible in some environmental units (for example, Dr Jean Munro's Brakespeare Hospital, near Watford) to have your levels of other chemical pollutants measured – e.g. heavy metals, petrol and petrochemical residues, insecticide and fertilizer by-products, etc. It is actually possible to have blood 'cleaned' of chemical pollutants by the use of intravenous drips of vitamin C. Another approach is chelation therapy, in which these toxins are 'bound' to safe chemicals given intravenously and then excreted in the urine. Chelation therapy is better known for its use to improve arteriosclerosis or narrowing of the arteries due to excessive fat intake and high stress levels.

Detoxification

Many therapeutic dietary processes start with a detoxification, or 'spring cleaning', regime. Using again the simple analogy of a machine, if you were to realize that the petrol you were putting in your car was full of sludge and contaminants, the first thing you would go about doing would be to decoke or clean the engine.

The body has three ways of dealing with dietary excess and impurity: to metabolize it (break it down), excrete it or deposit it in the tissues. When the excretory processes become overloaded, excess becomes deposited and our fat and body tissues become loaded up with chemical pollutants and partially digested metabolic by-products.

The detoxification process usually revolves around stopping or minimizing input to the body for a period of between a day and six weeks at the other extreme, in order to give the body an opportunity to complete the metabolic and excretion processes it would naturally be able to fulfil if it were not being continuously bombarded with more excess and impurity! For this reason, some people make detoxification on a regular basis part of their way of life. The most famous of these was Coco Chanel, who ate only fruit and drank only pure spring water every Sunday, and who put her luminous beauty down to the regular observation of this cleansing practice. Of course, if we eat a well-balanced diet all the time it should not be necessary to detox on a regular basis, but quite often where there has been a long-term poor eating pattern, or where an illness seems to be related to the way in which a person has been eating, detoxification can be an attractive starting place to give the body the best chance of getting back into a state of equilibrium.

There are all sorts of detoxification and fasting regimes, varying from taking pure water alone to fruit juices alone, to having just fruit juices and fruit. Others go for brown rice fasting, feeling that it is less stressful to the body (since it provides a constant supply of carbohydrate energy and vitamins to the system). In the more rigorous methods where only water and fruit juice are taken, you are not only cleaning the body but you are also putting it into starvation, which has other medical implications and makes the body hang on to things rather than let them go.

In some regimes the use of coffee enemas is advocated to enhance the detoxification process, as this has been found to increase the liver's excretory functions several fold. It is certainly noticeable that those using coffee enemas do become very bright-eyed and clear-skinned! This practice is much derided but is actually unanimously praised by those who have ever practised it.

Colonic irrigation

Another very mechanical form of detoxification is the practice of colonic irrigation, where the bowel is flooded with tepid normal saline and literally washed out. There are many extraordinary tales of the startling material which can be passed as a result of this process, where the bowel has become impacted with the results of years of low-fibre eating. As with hardening of the arteries, this waste material sticks to the wall of the bowel and greatly inhibits its function.

A cautionary note

Fasting and detoxification is a stressful process which should ideally be undergone with medical supervision. Sometimes detoxification regimes provoke what is known as a 'healing crisis'. This happens when the input of toxins ceases. Toxins can flood out of the tissues back into the bloodstream and can temporarily create quite an unpleasant toxic state. This can exacerbate symptoms for a while, sometimes quite dramatically, so it is ideal to have an experienced physician on hand to help you if necessary. Fasting is also inappropriate if you are already feeling very weak, toxic and vulnerable through illness or treatment. Unfortunately, it is while feeling ill that detoxification is often embarked upon as a last-ditch measure. It is advisable that your condition be reasonably stable before you take this sort of step.

Simple spring-cleaning diet

Having given all of these warnings, there is a middle path. Best known as a 'spring-cleaning diet', it entails putting yourself on a very clean, simple diet (comprised mainly of freshly made fruit juice, raw fruit, vegetables and salad, brown rice, cereals and lightly steamed vegetables) over a period of two to three months. In this way, without becoming hungry or having a strong detoxification crisis, you will very quickly clean out your system and feel very good indeed.

Cancer detox diets

There are many different sorts of detoxification diets specifically designed to be used to help the healing process in people who have been diagnosed as having cancer. The most famous for those with cancer are the Gerson diet, the Breuss Juice fast, the Kelly regime, grape fasting, Dr Moerman's diet and Dr Alec Forbes' Bristol Diet. In the Gerson diet, a very high-quality, organic, vegan, whole-food regime is combined with hourly freshly squeezed fruit and vegetable juices, and daily coffee enemas. As well as detoxification, the overall aim is to redress the body's sodium–potassium balance by providing a diet very low in sodium and high in potassium, with a view to restoring the natural vitality and 'electrical polarization' of cells. Recent evidence in favour of this theoretical approach has emerged, as the electrical polarization or 'transmembrane potential' of healthy cells has been found to be significantly higher than that of cancer cells. *(See Glossary for more about electrical polarization and transmembrane potential.)*

Raising Your Energy Level through Raw Foods

All the old complementary medical systems and exercise forms, such as acupuncture, shiatsu, homoeopathy, yoga and t'ai chi, are based around the idea that we have a vital force or energy system which is strong and balanced in good health and depleted and imbalanced in poor health. One of the ways that our vital force becomes chronically undermined is through eating foods which are themselves very low in life-force due to intensive farming, storage, cooking and processing techniques. It is therefore obvious that filling the body with very fresh, live, raw foods can have a significant effect on raising energy levels and improving the functioning of our tissues. This rise in energy occurs because raw, fresh foods have the highest level of vitamins, enzymes and phytochemicals, which are normally denatured by heating and storage processes. This is the underlying philosophy behind the approaches of Leslie Kenton in her raw-foods recipe books, and Ann Wigmore in her living-foods diet and approaches where wheat grass is juiced and taken along with a predominantly raw diet (as in the Hippocrates diet).

All of these approaches revolve around making raw fruit and vegetables (either whole or juiced) a very large proportion of one's diet. Anyone who has ever tried this will tell you that within a very short amount of time they feel absolutely wonderful (provided that they were not too weak, ill or underweight before they started the process). Inevitably, eating this way will also cause fairly rapid weight-loss, so it is very important to find a sustainable balance which includes enough protein, carbohydrates and fats if you are going to stay on a natural, predominantly raw, high-energy diet.

Correcting Nutritional Imbalances

While there are general nutritional rules and guidelines for healthy eating, it is never clearer than in the field of nutrition that each individual is unique. Foods and regimes that suit one person will not suit another. In fact, for some, dietary intolerance for certain foods and the resulting irritation to the bowel mucosa may be severe enough in their own right to start cancer. As described earlier, many diseases and conditions can have a strong nutritional component, so if you feel you may have a food-related disorder, such as an allergy or problems with digestion, it is very important to seek the advice of a nutritional therapist.

The hay diet

Many people have found relief from chronic digestive, acidity and absorption problems by adopting variations on the theme of the Hay diet. In this 'food combining' diet, the major focus is to eat either only proteins or only starches with your salad or vegetables at each meal. It is quite complex to follow, but there are excellent books around for guidance and it has certainly revolutionized wellbeing and made a very significant contribution to reducing the symptoms of diseases ranging from arthritis to angina!

Anti-candida diets

Diets to help clear up candida (thrush) in the intestines are always aimed at reducing intake of refined sugar, alcohol and sometimes yeast. Sometimes the individual is also advised to take either caprilic acid or another anti-fungal preparation. This often undiagnosed condition can create a great deal of malaise, fatigue and cloudy-headedness, as well as abdominal bloating. Receiving treatment for this condition can be like turning on a light after a long period in darkness!

Anti-allergy diets

Allergies or sensitivities to certain foods and environmental toxins are another source of a whole range of diverse symptoms. It is always a good idea to eliminate any foods to which you are allergic from your diet so you are not depleting your energy or diverting the attention of your immune system to dealing with the offending allergen. And again, a nutritional therapist could help you pinpoint those foods to which your body is sensitive.

Correcting Energetic Imbalances

As well as the Eastern therapeutic and exercise systems which relate to the energy balance or imbalance of the body, there is also a dietary approach which works on this level, namely macrobiotics. In complementary medicine systems which look at the energy function of the body, the energy is seen as having positive and negative polarities, just as in electrical circuitry. In macrobiotics, these two opposing qualities are known as *yin* and *yang*. The yin foods tend to be the sweeter, lighter foods, and the yang foods are heavier foods such as meat, eggs and cheese.

In a perfectly healthy individual, the aim would be to eat a diet where the yin and yang elements are completely balanced – so there are no 'forbidden' foods as such. However, to balance the eating of a 14-oz steak you would probably need to eat half a sack of brown rice! So once again we see that the basic guideline is to concentrate on the foods which are in the middle, between these two extremes, that is fruits, vegetables, soups, grains and cereals, in a ratio of:

grains and cereals 50–60 per cent

vegetables and fruits 25–30 per cent

protein as beans and soya products 5–10 per cent

soups 5 per cent.

This is extremely close to the current guidelines for healthy eating put forward by Western nutritional experts, in their understanding of the need for more fibre, fruits and vegetables without excessively high amounts of fat, protein, salt or sugar in the diet.

In somebody with a disease, however, the macrobiotic dietary therapist would be seeking to help correct the energy, or *chi*, imbalance by prescribing an individual macrobiotic diet, in which case the macrobiotic diet is definitely being used as a medicine or therapy.

As with all these dietary approaches there have been notable successes – and notable failures – so it is necessary to have expert advice, clear information and very good support before embarking on this approach.

Food as Medicine

The use of food as medicine comes under the broad heading of *naturopathy*.

Naturopathy is a very old, elegant and efficacious system of medicine. Many foods are known to have strong medicinal properties which can affect our mood states, heart rate and strength, digestive processes, liver functioning, tissue acidity and alkalinity, skin-healing ability – in fact, every level of our functioning.

In the last decade there has been a great deal of exciting medical research into the potential role of certain foods in the prevention and treatment of cancer. Some of the most promising research has been with green leafy vegetables and broccoli; yellow and orange vegetables such as yellow peppers and carrots; onions; and soya products. The cabbages and broccoli (and other plants in the brassica family) have been found to contain a compound called *indole-glycosinate*, which is anti-cancerous. This is available in tablet form as *Indole-3-Carbinol* from the Nutri-Centre in Regents Park in London. It has both a direct anti-cancer effect as well as an indirect anti-cancer effect on hormone-triggered cancers by channelling the production of oestrogen in the body into a metabolic pathway which results in the production of the least stimulatory form of oestrogen. It is being taken by some women with breast cancer as an alternative to the oestrogen-blocking drug, *Tamoxifen*. The yellow/orange vegetables have been found to contain a combination of factors – including betacarotene, calcium, selenium and micro-nutrients – which work in concert to produce a strong anti-cancer effect.

Soya products and fermented soya products such as miso have been found to contain phyto-oestrogens (plant oestrogens which block oestrogen activity, like the drug *Tamoxifen*), phytate, protease inhibitors, isoflavinoides and isoflavones, which are thought to be inhibitors of oncogenes – the part of the DNA in the cell and the chromosome in the cell nucleus which is thought to be responsible for setting off cancer cell growth and multiplication. Studies with miso have shown definite cancer-protective effects. Lemons contain limonene, and tomatoes lycopene, which are also anti-cancer agents; shitake mushrooms, kombu and kelp also interfere with the *initiation* and *promotion* of cancer cells *(see Glossary)*.

A very wide range of plant chemicals is being tested for their anti-cancer and healing properties. Substances collectively known as phytochemicals include plant phenols, aromatic isothiocyanates, methylated flavones, coumarines, plant sterols, as well as naturally occurring plant selenium salts, ascorbic acid (vitamin C) with its accompanying bioflavinoids and co-factors (now thought to be as important as the vitamin itself), tocopherols, retinols and carotenes. Many of these substances have been seen to act together to render carcinogenic substances harmless, and to repair damage to DNA and RNA in the cell's nucleus, thereby preventing tumour formation.

The protease inhibitors like those found in soy are thought to protect cells from ionizing radiation, including the X-rays used in cancer therapy.

Dietary fibre protects us in two ways: first through phytates and lignans, such as genistein and diadzein, which directly lower the production of free radicals; and by speeding up the transit time of carcinogens through the bowel, thereby decreasing their absorption and harmful effects. Specific anti-cancer effects have also been found for curcumin, the active ingredient in the Indian culinary herb turmeric.

The most authoritative work on this subject is Susannah Olivier's *The Breast Cancer Prevention and Recovery Diet*, from which the following table is reproduced with her permission. Further scientific references to the research done on the important anti-cancer phytochemicals can be found in her book for those who wish to take their studies further.

Anti-cancer foods and the phytochemicals they contain

FOOD	PHYTO-CHEMICAL
Alfalfa	Saponins, sterols, flavinoids, coumarins and alkaloids, various vitamins and minerals
Alliums: onions, spring onions, garlic, leeks, chives	Allium compounds diallyl sulfide and allyl methyl trisulphide
Almonds	Protease inhibitors, phytate, genistein, lignins and benzaldehyde
Apples	Chlorogenic acid and caffeic acid
Brassicas: broccoli, cabbage, Brussels sprouts, collards, kale, bok choy, kohl rabi, arugula, horseradish, radish, rutabagas and turnips	Dithiolthiones, isothiocyanates, glucosinolates, Indole-3-Carbinol and sulphurophane (in broccoli)

Sprouted Broccoli and cauliflower seeds	Sulphurophane (10–100 times higher than in the vegetables themselves)
Burdock Root (Gobo)– a component of the cancer remedy *Essiac*	Benzaldehyde, phytosterols, glycosides, mokko lactone and arctic acid
Citrus fruits	Counarins and hesperatin, narangenin, glutathione and bioflavinoids
Flaxseed oil	Omega-3 essential fatty acids and antioxidants
Garlic	Selenium, germanium, antioxidants, isoflavones and allyl sulphide
Ginger	Antioxidants, gingerol and carotenes
Grapes	Antioxidants and ellagic acid (raisins also contain tannins and caffeic acid)
Liquorice	Triterpenoids
Linseeds	Lignins and omega-3 fatty acids and alpha linolenic acid
Mushrooms (maitake, rei-shi, shiitake)	Polysaccharide immune stimulants (which boost interferon and interleukin levels), selenium, antioxidants, lignins and adaptogenic compounds
Nettles	Carotenes, chlorophyll, folic acid and selenium
Fresh nuts and seeds, particularly almonds, walnuts and black walnuts, pecans, sunflower seeds, sesame seeds and linseeds (flaxseeds)	Protease inhibitors, essential fats and antioxidant
Olive oil	Specific antioxidants

Orange/red/purple-coloured foods such as apricots, cantaloupe, carrots, yellow and red peppers, beets, squashes, sweet potatoes, red and black berries	Betacarotene and proanthocyanadins (amongst the most powerful antioxidants known)
Parsley	Phytosterols, carotenes, folic acid, chlorophyll, vitamin C, the essential oils terpenes, and pinenes and polyacetylene
Pineapple	Bromelain, protease inhibitors, citris, folic, malic and chlorogenic acids
Potatoes	Protease inhibitors, chlorogenic acid and vitamin C
Legumes and Beans	Protease inhibitors, lignins, genistein and phytosterols
Brown rice	Rice bran saccharide
Seaweeds: kombu, kelp, nori, arame, lava bread, dulse, wakame	Antioxidants, carotenes, selenium, iodine, alginic acid, the full range of minerals and trace elements and vitamin B12
Soy products	The isoflavones genistein and diadzein, phytic acid, saponins, phytosterols, protease inhibitors, omega-3 fatty acids and lecithin
Teas: Black tea	The polyphenols theaflavin and thearubigin (which interfere with the initiation, promotion and growth stages of cancer)
Green tea	Epicatechin (the strongest anti-mutagen of any plant yet examined) and epigallocatechin-3-gallate
All leaf teas	Anti-mutagenic tannins, antioxidants and polyphenols
Tomatoes	Antioxidants, flavinoids, lycopene, chlorogenic acid, coumarins, carotenes and caretenoids
Turmeric	Curcumin

The criticism aimed at many dietary therapeutic approaches for people who have cancer is that they can be very demanding in terms of time, energy and money, and can lead to relative social isolation as well as, potentially, to the tricky waters of the healing crisis *(see page 77)* and rapid weight loss. If these therapeutic approaches are embarked upon either to prevent or treat cancer, it is essential that this is done with adequate support, professional help and information.

Another problem is that therapeutic diets emerging from different colleges or schools of thought are often contradictory because of the differing underlying principles involved. The key here is to choose one approach and stick to it, not flit from one to another. However, with the emerging information about the specific factors within foods which may be protective, it is becoming possible (as with Indole-3-Carbinol and curcumin) to isolate the protective factors and incorporate them into extremely specific and effective anti-cancer regimes, thus avoiding some of the dogma and extremism of some of the dietary therapeutic approaches. It must be said that many people with cancer know that being positive and having a fighting spirit play a very important part in the recovery process, but it is impossible to be positive in a vacuum. Having an exacting dietary approach to follow can actually provide a framework for a self-help approach, and has for many people been an extremely important starting place on their healing journey, serving as a concrete symbol of their intention to do well and conquer the disease. Almost universally, this results in a great improvement in energy and vitality, which has made embarking upon other lifestyle changes much easier. At the same time, many who follow healthy-eating or detox diets have reported wonderful, unexpected side-benefits, such as the disappearance or dramatic improvement of long-standing skin, asthmatic or joint problems.

Food Supplementation with Vitamins and Minerals for the Treatment and Prevention of Cancer

Frequently the response to the suggestion that vitamins, minerals and essential nutrients form an important part of an anti-cancer diet is met with the comment, 'Why on earth do I need to take extra vitamins and minerals if I am going to be eating such a good diet?'

Certainly, eating well will exert a very large protective effect, but the issue here is that we are exposed to environmental pollution with petrochemicals, industrial by-products in our water systems, farming residues of pesticides and insecticides, and the effects of ionizing radiation and increased UV light, and as such are potentially exposed to destabilizing chemical influences which can trigger the cancer process. Until we are in a position to make a significant improvement in levels of pollution, it is wise to take some antioxidant vitamin and mineral protection.

In general terms, the reasons for taking extra vitamins and minerals are:

- replacement of long-term nutritional deficiencies
- boosting of immune function
- deactivating of dangerous free radicals and pollutants
- direct stabilization of cell membranes and cancer cells
- possible regulation of oncogene, thought to be associated with cancer cell growth
- for those with cancer who may be facing rigorous treatment, to compensate for the tissue loss caused by surgery, chemotherapy and radiotherapy.

The relevance of the use of vitamins and minerals for those with cancer was first taught to me by the Chief Medical Officer of Great Britain, Dr Kenneth Calman, when he was in charge of cancer services for the West of Scotland in 1985.

There are now thousands of high-quality, scientific, peer-reviewed studies providing solid evidence for the role of nutrition in cancer development, treatment and prevention. The body of research grows year by year, much of it now being carried out by the mainstream cancer charities – yet many doctors remain largely unaware of this huge body of work.

The use of vitamins and minerals in cancer-treatment protocols should now be routine, and all of us living in industrialized society would be well advised to take preventive vitamin and mineral supplementation.

Vitamins betacarotene, C, E and the mineral selenium given to 50,000 Chinese for five years brought down cancer deaths overall by 13 per cent, and death from their most common cancers by 20 per cent.[1]

Some doctors feel that the doses of vitamins being given are very high, but these are based on levels which have been found in hundreds of trials to produce the best results. It must be remembered that most of the recommended daily dosages of these substances taught to doctors in medical schools are the amounts needed to prevent deficiency diseases such as rickets and scurvy. Clearly, at this time we are looking at a very different set of demands on the human body due to the evolution and 'civilization' of society, which necessitates taking much higher levels of these substances. In fact, most mammals other than man have retained the ability to synthesize vitamin C themselves, and synthesize it at the sort of level that would be equivalent to our taking the recommended 3–6 grams per day.

Vitamins and minerals in adequate quantities are essential to health. They are needed by the immune system, and some may play a more direct part in protecting the body against cancer. Stress, illness and its treatment increase the body's need for supplements of this kind, and studies have shown that people who have developed cancer can have relatively low levels of these essential substances. It makes sense, then, to ensure that the body is not allowed to develop a state of vitamin and mineral deficiency, particularly as many people also report that they cope better with radiotherapy and chemotherapy when they are taking supplements. This is backed by scientific studies.[2]

Retinoids (vitamin A) and betacarotene (vitamin A precursor) have been shown to have very powerful anti-cancer effects, even returning cancer cells back towards normal in laboratory conditions.[3] Low vitamin A levels are linked with cancer of the colon, lung, cervix, larynx, bladder, oesophagus, stomach, rectum, prostate and mouth.[4] Paradoxically, however, recent studies have shown that smokers who take betacarotene may be at *increased* risk of cancer. Obviously, I would suggest giving up the cigarettes rather than the betacarotene![5]

Hundreds of studies of vitamin C have shown a preventive effect on cancer.[6] Vitamin C is the fastest free-radical scavenger and can also boost our oxygen supply by improving the blood's haemoglobin status. Its effectiveness can be enhanced by vitamin K and chelated iron.

Stress lowers our vitamin C levels, which is yet another reason why stress leaves us so vulnerable. Low levels of vitamin C have been found in people with cancer of the uterus, cervix and ovary, and in those with leukaemia and lymphoma.[7]

Vitamin E is also antioxidant, and helps the body to make proper use of the mineral selenium, especially when taken in the natural tocopherol form (rather than as the synthetic succinate). Selenium is itself a preventive or resistance factor in cancer, as it protects against free radicals, mutagens, toxic heavy metals and certain bacterial, viral and fungal agents which cause disease.[8]

Vitamin C (as calcium or magnesium ascorbate)

Start with 500mg 3 times daily, and increase gradually to 2g 3 times daily or take 500mg of Nature's Own Food State vitamin C, 3 times daily

Please note: If you get an upset stomach, reduce the dose and stick to the level which does not cause diarrhoea. The ascorbic acid form is best avoided as this can be too acidic, causing stomach upsets at lower levels.

Betacarotene

15mg capsule once daily, or 3 x 5mg tablets once daily (approximately 25,000iu daily). Half a pint of carrot juice is equivalent to 5mg or 10,000iu, so reduce tablet dose accordingly if taking juice. (Betacarotene is the safe form in which to take vitamin A.)

Please note: Betacarotene is a pigment and may occasionally cause the skin to turn orange. If this happens, reduce dose but do not worry. The staining of the skin will not harm you, and will soon fade as levels drop.

Selenium

200mg daily

Vitamin E

400iu daily

Please note: Historically there is some controversy over the use of vitamin E in hormone-dependent cancers (that is, breast, uterus, ovarian, prostate and testicular), as it may boost hormone levels. However, evidence for the benefits of vitamin E in these cancers now far outweighs theoretical concerns to the contrary and its use for people with hormonal cancers is now recommended.

Vitamin B complex

50mg daily
B complex contains all of the B vitamins in one tablet.

Please note: This may turn your urine bright yellow, but there is no need to be concerned about this.

Zinc orotate (or gluconate)
100mg daily, or zinc citrate 50mg daily or 15mg of elemental zinc
Reduce after 3 months to 30mg zinc orotate (15mg zinc citrate) daily (approximately 5mg elemental zinc) as zinc can begin to accumulate in the body.

Please note: Zinc is not well absorbed so it is best not taken with food; this can easily be achieved by taking it last thing at night.

FOR PREVENTION OF CANCER AND FOR THOSE IN REMISSION FROM CANCER

Vitamin C	1g 3 times daily or 250mg Nature's Own Food State vitamin C, 3 times daily
Betacarotene	15mg daily (25,000iu)
Selenium	200mcg daily
Vitamin E	400iu
Zinc orotate	30mg daily (elemental zinc 5mg daily)
Vitamin B complex	50mg daily

VITAMINS AND MINERALS DURING RADIOTHERAPY AND CHEMOTHERAPY
Vitamin C augments the effectiveness of radiotherapy and can help decrease the anaemia, pain, appetite loss and weight loss experienced by those on this form of treatment. It protects the heart for those on the chemotherapeutic drug Adriamycin (as does co-enzyme Q10 or Ubiquinone).[9] Vitamin C also enhances the effectiveness of chemotherapeutic agents 5-Fluo-uracil and Bleomycin. Vitamin E reduces cardiac and skin toxicity and hair loss for those on Doxorubicin, protects lymph tissue against Bleomycin, and decreases cardio-toxicity of Adriamycin. Betacarotene potentiates the effectiveness of 5-Fluo-uracil, Methotrexate and Cobalt therapy. Selenium is also radio- and chemo-protective, and protects the kidneys against cisplatin. Radiotherapy decreases levels of vitamin E, B12, folic acid and C, so it is a good idea to ensure either a diet rich in these substances or supplementation while on radiotherapy.[10]

Remedies During Chemotherapy

For abdominal disturbances, take aloe vera juice (1 tbs 3 times a day); or slippery elm powder (1 tsp 3 times a day) in a concentrated herb tea or mixed with soya milk or yoghurt; or comfrey tea (3 times per day). Slippery elm can also be taken as a tablet 3 times a day.

For Nausea

Try root ginger, grated or as a tea (also available as tea bags). Some people also find sea-bands useful: these are bands worn on the wrist and are marketed for use against seasickness. They work by exerting pressure on relevant acupuncture points through little pads, and are remarkably effective. Most chemists stock them. Slippery elm is also often useful for nausea.

Remedies During Radiotherapy

The side-effects of radiotherapy may be helped by Homoeopathic Radiation Remedy (obtainable from Galen Homoeopathics, Lewell Mill, West Stafford, near Dorchester). Aloe vera and vitamin E cream or Louise Brackenbury's Aromatherapy Radiation Cream (obtainable from the shop at Bristol Cancer Help Centre) may be used to protect your skin during and after radiotherapy.

Problems Swallowing Pills and Capsules

Many vitamins can be obtained in droplet form. Most tablets can be crushed and capsules pierced to make them palatable by mixing them in fruit juice or soup.

Problems with Absorption

If you suspect, for whatever reason, that you may have a problem absorbing vitamins, you might consider using sub-lingual products, designed to be absorbed under the tongue or in the cheek cavity.

Coenzyme Q10 or Ubiquinone

This substance is receiving a great deal of attention as a potential protection and treatment in cancer. It forms part of the energy-producing mechanism in cells, and has an antioxidant function. In a Danish study of women with breast cancer, many women experienced pronounced improvement of their condition. In the study, the women took up to 300mg per day.[11] For prevention purposes, 90mg per day would be ample.

A Final Thought

I hope that you will now feel sufficiently convinced, informed and inspired to set about changing the way you eat, confident that this can cause a really good creative and exciting change in your life and health. I hope that you feel encouraged to make the change in a gentle, exploratory way without stressing yourself or making yourself unhappy in the process.

Jane Sen, nutrition consultant and chef, and the author of the delicious recipes in this book, has demonstrated beyond a shadow of a doubt that vegan cookery can be just as accessible, mouth-watering and glamorous as any other form of food.

Play, experiment and become convinced of the real potential for delighting yourself with this way of cooking and eating, and enjoy the satisfaction and deep healing process which comes from properly nurturing yourself as you become fit, healthy, happy and strong.

The Recipes

Breakfasts

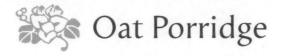

Oat Porridge

A wonderfully nourishing and inexpensive start to any day. Try this with any of the suggested porridge toppings (see page 97) or experiment with your own favourites. An even creamier version can be produced using a double saucepan (boiler); it takes a little longer to cook but the results are worth it.

SERVES 2

1 cup rolled or porridge oats
2 cups water

Bring to the boil in a heavy pan (non-stick saves washing-up tears). Reduce the heat and simmer very gently for approximately 15 minutes until thick and creamy (the time will depend on the thickness of your oats). Stir once or twice during cooking.

Serve with a splash of soya, oat or rice milk.

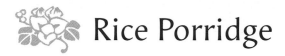

Rice Porridge

This porridge will keep for a couple of days in the fridge and can be reheated or served cold.

SERVES 4

approx. 115g (4oz/½ cup) whole brown rice
approx. 850ml (1½ pints/3¾ cups) soya milk

Combine in an electric slow-cooker pot and cook on the lowest setting overnight. In the morning you will have a delicious, creamy and nourishing bowl of delight.

Enjoy as it is or try any combination of toppings *(see below)*.

SUGGESTIONS FOR PORRIDGE TOPPINGS

- Maple syrup
- Date syrup
- Sesame seeds, roasted or not
- Flaxseeds (linseeds)
- Chopped dried fruits such as apricots, dates, prunes, figs, sultanas, raisins
- Sliced fresh banana
- Breakfast fruit compote *(see recipe on page 102)*
- Stewed dessert apples or plums

Crunchy Granola Breakfast Cereal

6 tablespoons honey
1 tablespoon olive oil

Warm together and stir into:

455g (1lb/5 cups) rolled or porridge oats

Turn onto a large baking sheet or roasting tray, spread evenly and loosely and place in a preheated oven to crisp up. Stir and turn regularly until evenly toasted and beginning to turn golden.

115g (4oz/⅘ cup) chopped or whole almonds
115g (4oz /1 cup) sunflower seeds
55g (2oz/½ cup) sesame seeds

Gently roast and toast in a heavy, dry pan, stirring continuously until they release their nutty aroma. Add to crunchy oat mixture and allow to cool.

A couple of handfuls of dried fruits such as sultanas and raisins may be added at this stage before storing in an airtight container. If you want your granola to stay really crunchy, just sprinkle on the fruits each time you serve as the moisture in the fruits can sometimes begin to soften the mix if storing for a longer period.

Serve with soya, rice or oat milk.

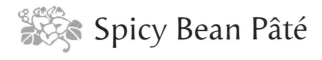

Spicy Bean Pâté

225g (8oz/ 1½ cups) pinto or aduki beans, soaked overnight
4 garlic cloves, peeled

Cook the beans with the garlic in water until the beans are very soft. When cooked, mash with a fork or whizz in a blender.

1 large onion, finely chopped
2 garlic cloves, crushed (minced)
1 red or green pepper (bell pepper), finely chopped
2 tablespoons olive oil
1 teaspoon ground cumin
1 teaspoon paprika
2 teaspoons tamari

Sauté the vegetables in the oil over a gentle heat until soft. Stir in the spices. Fry for another few minutes then add the tamari. Stir the vegetable mixture into the beans and press into 6 ramekin pots or a bowl. Cool.

Boston Baked Beans

Be sure to make plenty as the beans freeze well in individual portions.

900g (2lb/4½ cups) haricot or small white beans

Cook in simmering water until soft (approx. 1 ½–2 hours), drain and set aside.

2 onions, finely chopped
4 tablespoons olive oil
2 teaspoons oregano
1 teaspoon marjoram

In a heavy pan, sauté together until the onions are soft, then add:

3 teaspoons tomato purée (tomato paste)

and stir and sizzle for a few more minutes. Then add:

455g (1lb/2 cups) chopped fresh or tinned tomatoes
2 tablespoons malt extract
2 cups water
ground black or cayenne pepper to taste
2 tablespoons tamari soy sauce

Simmer for about 10 minutes. Whizz till smooth in a goblet blender or with a hand blender. Add the beans and cook very gently for a further 20–30 minutes. Serve on wholemeal (whole-wheat) toast.

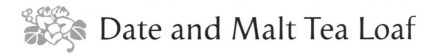

Date and Malt Tea Loaf

Sticky and tasty, this loaf gets better and better on keeping.

570ml (1 pint/2½ cups) weak tea such as Earl Grey
455g (1lb/3 cups) pitted dates

Simmer gently for approximately 20 minutes until the dates are soft. Mash until the liquid is absorbed.

225g (8oz/1 cup) malt extract (malt syrup)
2 tablespoons date syrup

Add to the date mixture and allow to cool a little.

225g (8oz / 1½ cups) wholemeal (whole-wheat) flour
115g (4oz/scant 1 cup) organic white flour
1 teaspoon ground ginger
1 teaspoon ground nutmeg
1 teaspoon ground mixed spice (apple pie spice)

Sift into a large bowl and quickly and thoroughly stir into the date mixture. Turn into a greased and lined 900g/2lb loaf pan and bake in the oven for 40 minutes. Lower the heat and continue cooking for a further 20 minutes. Cool in the pan, remove and wrap tightly. Store overnight before slicing to serve.

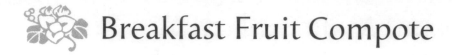

Breakfast Fruit Compote

There are endless variations on this sweet treat – you will find your own favourites but here is a good basic start. It keeps well in the fridge for a few days.

SERVES 4

115g (4oz/½ cup) dried unsulphured apricots
115g (4oz/½ cup) dried prunes
115g (4oz/⅔ cup) dried apple or pear slices
115g (4oz/⅘ cup) dried dates
water or apple juice to cover

In a heavy pan, bring to the boil, reduce the heat, cover and simmer slowly for approximately 30 minutes until all the fruits are really soft and the juices rich and syrupy. Serve warm or cold.

Light Lunches

Fresh Corn Chowder

If you blend the whole lot until smooth, this becomes a versatile sauce for pouring over other cooked vegetables. You can also layer it with slices of parboiled potatoes, bake at 190°C/375°F/Gas Mark 5 for 35–40 minutes and you'll have a tasty lunch dish to serve with a salad.

SERVES 4–6

3 tablespoons olive or sunflower oil
2 medium onions, finely chopped

In a large pan, sauté over a low heat for 8 minutes.

4 fresh corn cobs
1 potato, finely chopped
570ml (1 pint/2 ½ cups) soya milk
570ml (1 pint/2½ cups) water or vegetable stock
2 teaspoons low-salt stock (bouillon) powder
1 teaspoon ground black pepper
½ teaspoon ground nutmeg

Discard the leaves and hairy bits of the corn cobs. For each, stand the fat end firmly on a large chopping board, hold the pointed end and use a sharp knife to cut straight down behind the kernels to remove them from the cob.

Stir the corn and the rest of the ingredients into the onion mixture and gently bring to the boil. Simmer gently for 35 minutes.

Remove from the heat and allow to cool slightly. Blend half the soup in a blender and return to the pan. Heat gently again and serve.

Creamy Cauliflower Soup

2 medium potatoes, scrubbed and chopped (if you
want a really smooth soup, peel them first)
570ml (1 pint/2 ½ cups) soya milk
570ml (1 pint/2 ½ cups) vegetable stock or water
4 teaspoons low-salt stock (bouillon) powder

Simmer together gently, covered, in a large pan until the potatoes are really soft.

1 medium cauliflower, cut into small pieces (include stalks and small leaves)
handful of fresh mint leaves or 2 teaspoons dried mint
1 teaspoon ground nutmeg
1 teaspoon ground black pepper
4 sprigs of fresh mint, to garnish

Add these ingredients to the pan and simmer, uncovered, for approximately 20 minutes, until the cauliflower is tender.

Let the mixture cool slightly and blend until smooth – not for too long or the potatoes can become gluey. Serve with a sprig of mint on each bowl.

Warm Red Cabbage Salad
with Watercress and Toasted Pecans

1 small red cabbage, very finely shredded
2 small red onions, finely sliced and pulled into rings
55g (2oz/1 cup) watercress

Mix together gently and arrange on individual serving plates.

55g (2oz/½ cup) pecans or walnuts
2 tablespoons olive oil
1 small onion, very finely chopped
2 tablespoons orange juice
1 teaspoon finely grated orange rind (peel)
1 tablespoon cider vinegar

Sauté the nuts in half the oil until they are just turning golden. Remove with a slotted spoon and share out over the prepared salads.

Add the onion and remaining oil to the pan and stir over quite a high heat for a minute or two. Add the orange juice, boil for a minute, then stir in the other ingredients and heat through briefly. Pour over the salads and serve immediately.

Indonesian Sprout and Nut Salad

This salad is delicious on its own, or when quickly stirred into hot brown rice. Raw vegetables and hot grains make a wonderful one-bowl lunch.

SERVES 4–6

2 tablespoons light tahini
1 tablespoon roasted sesame oil (optional)
1 green chilli pepper, finely chopped (optional)
juice of 1 lemon
2 teaspoons tamari soy sauce
4 fresh mint leaves, finely chopped
2 tablespoons peanut butter
pinch of ground black pepper
little splash of cider vinegar

In a large salad bowl, combine to a smooth dressing.

115g (4oz/¾ cup) plain peanuts or cashews

In a dry pan, fry over a moderate heat until they begin to turn golden. Or roast them on a baking (cookie) sheet in the oven. Add to the dressing while still warm.

½ cucumber, finely chopped or grated
3–4 handfuls mung bean sprouts or chickpea (garbanzo bean) sprouts or your favourite mixture
2–3 radishes, finely chopped or grated
some chopped fresh coriander (cilantro) (optional)

Gently toss into the nuts and dressing and serve immediately. Sprinkle with fresh coriander (cilantro) if you can.

Broccoli, Macadamia and Garlic Salad

This is one of those recipes where having a few leftover cooked chickpeas (garbanzo beans)
in the refrigerator or freezer means you can make a very quick, tasty meal at the last
minute.

SERVES 4–6

approx. 85g (3oz/½ cup) cooked chickpeas (garbanzo beans)
2 tablespoons olive oil
90ml (3fl oz/⅓ cup) cider vinegar
2 garlic cloves
½ teaspoon ground black pepper

Combine for a few seconds in a blender until the mixture is the consistency of single
(light) cream. Add a little water or lemon juice if it's a bit thick.

2 or 3 fresh firm heads of broccoli, divided into florets and sliced from stem to top,
very thinly
140g (5oz/1 cup) macadamia nuts, sliced, or 65g (2½oz/½ cup) toasted pine
nuts

Pile the broccoli onto a plate or into a shallow bowl. Scatter with the nuts and drizzle
the dressing over the top.

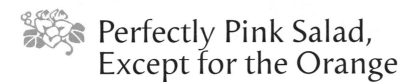

Perfectly Pink Salad, Except for the Orange

455g (1lb/8 cups) red cabbage, very finely shredded
1 tablespoon tamari soy sauce
1 tablespoon cider vinegar

Place in a large bowl and scrunch and knead together with your hand for a few minutes. Set aside.

2 apple-size beetroots, raw or cooked, peeled and grated
zest of 1 orange
large oranges, skin and pith removed with a sharp knife and flesh sliced
10–12 radishes, grated or thinly sliced
2 tablespoons olive oil (optional)
½ teaspoon ground black pepper

Gently combine with the cabbage mixture and allow to stand for a few minutes before serving. You can serve this on a bed of mixed green leaves but include watercress for extra nutrients if you can.

Spinach and Sunflower Seed Salad

Shredded red-skinned apple looks very pretty in this. Sunflower seeds prepared in this way keep very well in an airtight jar and are useful for sprinkling and snacking.

SERVES 4–6

140ml (¼ pint/⅔ cup) cider vinegar
2 tablespoons lemon juice
115g (4oz/½ cup) dried apricots

Bring the vinegar just to the boil in a small pan, remove from the heat and add the lemon juice and apricots. Leave to soak for about 30 minutes, stirring occasionally. Then drain over a bowl, reserving the juice. Chop the apricots.

140g (5oz/1 cup) sunflower seeds
2 tablespoons tamari

Put the seeds in a heavy, dry frying pan and stir gently over a medium heat until just turning golden. Remove from the heat and quickly mix in the tamari – it will sizzle a lot and go sticky. Immediately pour the mixture from the pan onto a cool plate or a sheet of greaseproof paper (wax paper).

680g (1½ lb/12 cups)   young leaf spinach, torn into bite-size
                               pieces

Put the spinach into a serving bowl and add the chopped apricots.

2 tablespoons olive oil   reserved juice from the apricots
1 teaspoon coarsely ground black
   pepper

Whisk together. Add to the spinach, apricots and sunflower seeds. Combine gently and serve.

Cucumber in Creamy Mint Dressing

As well as being refreshing and tasty, this dressing is a good example of how protein can be found in unexpected places in this style of healthy eating.

SERVES 4–6

half a cucumber, peeled and chopped
170g (6oz/⅔ cup) plain silken tofu
zest of ½ a lemon
juice of 2 lemons
2 teaspoons light tahini
2 teaspoons cider vinegar
½ teaspoon ground black pepper
handful of fresh mint leaves or 2 teaspoons dried mint

Whizz together in a blender till smooth.

1 large cucumber, grated or thinly sliced
4 tomatoes, finely chopped
sprigs of fresh mint, to garnish

Mix into the dressing and decorate with mint sprigs to serve.

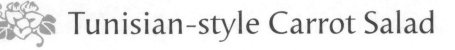# Tunisian-style Carrot Salad

85ml (3fl oz/scant ½ cup) oil
2 garlic cloves, very thinly sliced
450g (1lb) carrots, scrubbed and cut into thin strips

Heat the oil and toss in the carrots and garlic. Let sizzle for 2 minutes. Reduce the heat, cover and cook for 3-5 minutes more.

2 tablespoons cider vinegar
4 spring onions (scallions), sliced
½ teaspoon ground cloves
½ teaspoon ground cumin seeds
½ teaspoon paprika
1 teaspoon tamari

Add these to the pan in this order. Stir well, then remove from the heat.

2 tablespoons chopped fresh mint
a few sprigs of mint, to garnish

Add to the carrots. Transfer to a bowl and chill before serving, garnished with sprigs of mint.

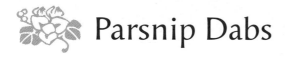

Parsnip Dabs

A really green vegetable, such as broccoli or curly kale, is the natural partner to these tasty morsels. Apple sauce goes well with them too.

MAKES APPROXIMATELY 12–14
OVEN: 190°C/375°F/GAS MARK 5

680g (1½lb/4 cups) parsnips, scrubbed and diced (peel them if they seem a bit tough or elderly)

Boil in water until soft (approximately 15 minutes). Drain and mash – don't worry if there are a few lumps.

1 tablespoon olive oil
2 teaspoons dried or fresh tarragon
1 medium onion, finely chopped

Fry gently in the oil until the onion is very soft. Combine with the mashed parsnips.

55g (2oz/½ cup) finely chopped walnuts
1 tablespoon tamari
1 teaspoon ground black pepper
2 tablespoons soya flour or rice flour

Mix well into the parsnips and onions. Allow to cool.

225g (8oz/2 cups) soft brown breadcrumbs

Divide the parsnip mixture into approximately 12 balls (each about the size of a large golf ball). Wetting your hands helps with this process. Roll the balls around, one by one, in the breadcrumbs and gently press onto an oiled baking sheet. If you have any crumbs left over, pat them onto the tops of the 'dabs'. Bake for 20 minutes.

Grilled (Broiled) Aubergines (Eggplant) with Salsa Verde

2 medium aubergines (eggplant), cut lengthways into 5mm (¼-inch) slices
4 tablespoons olive oil

Brush the slices with a little oil and grill (broil) on both sides until golden brown and soft (8–10 minutes).

2 garlic cloves, peeled and roughly chopped
2 tablespoons fresh parsley
2 tablespoons fresh basil
2 tablespoons pine nuts or almonds
½ teaspoon ground black pepper
100ml (3½]fl oz/scant ½ cup) olive oil

Place in a blender and process to a smoothish paste.

2 large tomatoes, finely chopped

Layer the aubergine (eggplant) slices alternately with the tomatoes. Pour over the salsa. Serve warm or chilled with hot bread, rice or couscous.

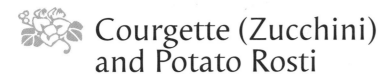

Courgette (Zucchini) and Potato Rosti

SERVES 4–6

3 medium potatoes, skins left on, coarsely grated
1 courgette (zucchini), grated
1 teaspoon ground black pepper
1 teaspoon black poppy seeds
pinch of fresh thyme leaves
1 tablespoon rice flour

Mix together well, then leave for 10 minutes before squeezing the liquid out firmly – twisting the mixture in a clean tea towel (dishcloth) is quite effective.

3 tablespoons olive oil
1 teaspoon tamari

Heat the oil in a heavy frying pan (skillet), preferably non-stick. Put the potato mixture in the pan and press carefully to an even thickness. Cook gently, without stirring or covering, for 20 minutes.

Turn the rosti over. This is considerably easier if you have another oiled pan to place over the top into which you can carefully invert the whole thing. If not, use an oiled plate and slide the turned rosti back into the same pan. Cook gently for 15–20 minutes more. Sprinkle with the tamari, slice and serve hot.

Spicy Oven Fries

Try serving these with a creamy soup for a delicious change to the usual soup accompaniments.

SERVES 4–6

OVEN: 200°C/400°F/GAS MARK 6

2 tablespoons olive oil
1 tablespoon tomato purée (tomato paste)
1 teaspoon paprika
1 tablespoon tamari
1 teaspoon ground black pepper

Whisk together in a large mixing bowl.

3 or 4 large potatoes, scrubbed and cut into fairly fat 'fingers' (approximately 12–14 from each potato)

Toss the potato fingers in the mixture, making sure they are evenly covered.
Turn into a roasting tin and bake for 35–40 minutes, until soft in the middle and a bit crunchy around the edges.

Chinese-style Stir-fried Vegetables

SERVES 4–6

3 tablespoons sunflower oil
1 teaspoon roasted sesame oil
15g (½oz) fresh ginger root,
    peeled and finely grated

1 large onion, sliced vertically
3 garlic cloves, finely grated
3 star anise (optional)

Heat the oil in a large wok. Toss in the onion and other ingredients and cook until just softened. Keep them on the move while you add your choice of the following selection – 3 or 4 work best. (Those at the top of the list need the longest cooking time so put them in first and stir for a minute or two before adding your other choices.)

2 carrots, very thinly sliced diagonally
1 head of broccoli, very thinly sliced
2 celery sticks, thinly sliced diagonally
1 green or red pepper (bell pepper), thinly sliced
4 medium mushrooms, sliced
10 button mushrooms, halved
170g (6oz/2 cups) mixed wild mushrooms
30g (1oz/¼ cup) dry arame or hijiki seaweed (soaked for 10 minutes
    in hot water)
115g (4oz/2 cups) shredded cabbage
115g (4oz/2 cups) shredded Chinese greens
115g (4oz/2 cups) mung bean sprouts

Toss around in the wok over quite a fierce heat until everything is heated through.

3 tablespoons tamari
3 tablespoons sesame seeds, to garnish

Pour the tamari over the mixture. Sprinkle with sesame seeds and serve with rice.

Good All Round Tomato Sauce

Great on any kind of pasta or vegetables. Left to reduce and thicken, it's a good pizza topping too.

MAKES ABOUT 1.2 LITRES (2 PINTS/5 CUPS)

4 tablespoons olive oil
2 onions, finely chopped
1 teaspoon dried oregano
1 teaspoon dried basil
1 teaspoon fennel seeds (optional)
4 garlic cloves, sliced
1 teaspoon ground black pepper

Soften together in a good, heavy-based saucepan.

115g (4oz/½ cup) tomato purée (tomato paste)
1 carrot, grated
1 small red or green pepper (bell pepper), finely chopped
395g (14oz/2 cups) chopped fresh or canned tomatoes
1 tablespoon tamari
285ml (½ pint/1⅓ cups) water
1 tablespoon dark malt extract

Stir the tomato purée (tomato paste) into the softened onion over a gentle heat for 3–4 minutes, then add the rest of the ingredients. Stir well, lower the heat and simmer for 25–30 minutes. Cook a little longer if you like it a bit thicker.

Orange and Sesame Dressing

Delicious on a mixture of finely shredded red and green cabbage, with sultanas and almonds.

zest (finely grated rind) of 1 large orange, the segments chopped
1 tablespoon cider vinegar
1 tablespoon tamari
1 teaspoon toasted sesame oil
1 teaspoon sesame seeds
2 tablespoons olive oil

Whizz together in a blender.

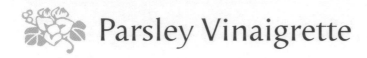

Parsley Vinaigrette

Vary this by using other herbs: basil is heavenly; mint or tarragon are good variations, too; or try a mixture with (or without) a clove of garlic.

140 ml (¼ pint/⅔ cup) olive oil
4 tablespoons cider vinegar
2 tablespoons tamari
1 teaspoon light tahini
zest (finely grated rind) of 1 lemon
55g (2oz/1 cup) fresh parsley

Whizz for a couple of minutes in a blender.

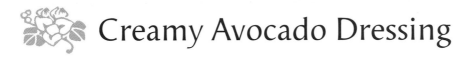

Creamy Avocado Dressing

2 ripe avocados, peeled and stone (pit) removed
300ml (½ pint/⅓ cup) soya milk
1 tablespoon tamari
juice of 1 lemon
pinch of paprika
1 teaspoon light tahini
pinch of ground black pepper

Blend until smooth.

Main Meals

FOR 225G (8OZ/1 CUP) DRY WEIGHT OF GRAIN.

GRAIN TYPE	WATER	SIMMERING TIME	APPROX. YIELD
Barley	3 cups / 24 fl oz / 750ml	1¼ hours	3½ cups / 28oz / 800g
Buckwheat	2 cups / 16 fl oz / 500ml	15 minutes	2½ cups / 20oz / 575g
Bulgar wheat, chewy	Soak in 4 cups / 32 fl oz / 1 litre hot water (to cover)	Drain after 30 minutes (no cooking)	2¼ cups / 18oz / 500g
Bulgar wheat, soft	2 cups / 16 fl oz / 500ml	15 minutes	2½ cups / 20oz / 575g
Couscous	Soak in 3 cups / 24 fl oz / 750ml	Steam or bake 10 minutes	2¼ cups / 18oz / 500g
Millet	3 cups / 24 fl oz / 750ml	35–40 minutes	3½ cups / 28oz / 800g
Quinoa	2 cups / 16 fl oz / 500ml	15 minutes	2½ cups / 20oz / 575g
Rice, brown or basmati	1½ cups / 12 fl oz / 375ml	25 minutes	2¼ cups / 18oz / 500g
Rice, brown – short or long grain	2 cups / 16 fl oz / 500ml	45 minutes	3 cups / 24oz / 675g
Whole-wheat berries	3 cups / 24 fl oz / 750ml	2 hours	2½ cups / 20oz / 575g
Wild rice	3 cups / 24 fl oz / 750ml	45–50 minutes	4 cups / 32oz / 900g

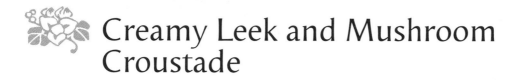

Creamy Leek and Mushroom Croustade

Lovely with Creamed Garlic Potatoes (page 132) and broccoli or a green salad.

SERVES 4–6
OVEN: 230°C/450°F/GAS MARK 8

30g (1oz) soya margarine
115g (4oz/2 cups) soft
   brown breadcrumbs
55g (2oz/⅔ cup) finely
   chopped almonds

2 tablespoons olive oil
115g (4oz/⅔ cup) ground
   hazelnuts
1 teaspoon tarragon
2 garlic cloves, crushed

Melt the margarine and oil together and mix thoroughly with the other ingredients. Press into a greased ovenproof cake tin or flan dish. Use the back of a spoon to press it down firmly. Bake for 15 minutes.

2 leeks, finely chopped
2 tablespoons olive oil
1 teaspoon ground nutmeg
285ml (½ pint/1⅓ cups)
   soya milk
1 tablespoon tamari

115g (4oz /1 cup) sliced mushrooms
1 teaspoon ground black pepper
55g (2oz/½ cup) wholemeal
   (whole-wheat) or rice flour
1 tablespoon olive oil

Sauté the leeks and mushrooms in the oil with the pepper and nutmeg. Cover and cook over a low heat for 10 minutes. Stir in the flour and slowly add the milk, stirring all the time. Simmer gently to thicken. Spoon the mixture onto the croustade base. Splash the top with a little olive oil and tamari and return to the oven for about 10 minutes.

Ginger and Sesame Carrots

*Fresh parsley or coriander (cilantro) is delicious stirred in just before serving. Finely
shredded raw spinach or chard leaves also go well with this and should be added at the
last minute. As a quick snack, this is scrumptious stuffed into warm, brown pitta bread
with a drizzle of light tahini and tamari.*

SERVES 4–6

3 tablespoons olive or sunflower oil
30g (1oz/¼ cup) sesame seeds
30g (1oz/¼ cup) fresh root ginger, peeled and grated
2 garlic cloves, grated (optional)
6 medium carrots, scrubbed and cut into matchsticks or thin diagonal slices

Heat the oil and sesame seeds together in a wok or an enamelled iron casserole.
When the seeds begin to pop, add the ginger and garlic (if using), and stir. Add the
carrots and stir well. Lower the heat a little, cover and cook for 6–10 minutes, stirring
once during this time.

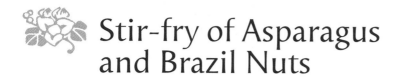

Stir-fry of Asparagus and Brazil Nuts

Serve with rice or buckwheat noodles.

SERVES 4–6

1 tablespoon arrowroot or cornflour (cornstarch)
2 tablespoons water
1 tablespoon tamari
1 tablespoon miso
140 ml (¼ pint/⅔ cup) water

Mix the arrowroot or cornflour (cornstarch) with the first measure of water until smooth, then blend with the other ingredients to form a smooth paste.

2 tablespoons sunflower oil
1 leek or onion, thinly sliced
1 tablespoon grated fresh root ginger
3 garlic cloves, grated
455g (1lb/3 cups) fresh asparagus spears,
    sliced diagonally into 2.5cm (1-inch) lengths
115g (4oz/1 cup) Brazil nuts, sliced
2 teaspoons toasted sesame seeds

Heat the oil in a wok over quite a high heat. Toss in the leek or onion, ginger and garlic. Stir and cook for 2 minutes, then add the asparagus and nuts. Stir and cook for 5 more minutes.

Pour in the miso mixture. Stir, reduce the heat and cook until the asparagus is just tender.

Sprinkle with the sesame seeds.

Moroccan-style Braised Vegetables and Butter Beans

4 tablespoons olive oil
1 or 2 cinnamon sticks

2 teaspoons fennel seeds
3 teaspoons dried oregano

Heat the oil gently with the fennel seeds, cinnamon and oregano in a deep roasting tin or casserole.

4 garlic cloves, sliced
1 teaspoon ground cloves
  or 6 whole cloves
2 teaspoons low-salt stock
  (bouillon) powder

3 onions, cut into fat wedges
2 teaspoons ground cinnamon
1 teaspoon ground nutmeg
1 teaspoon ground black pepper

Soften the garlic and onions a little in the herby oil, then add the spices and stock (bouillon) powder. Cook and stir for a few more minutes.

455g (1lb/3 cups) butternut or
  sweet orange-fleshed squash or
  sweet potato, cut into 2.5cm
  (1-inch) slices or chunky dice

455g (1lb/3 cups) carrots, scrubbed
  and cut lengthways into 4

455g (1lb/2 cups) cooked butter
  (lima) beans or chickpeas
  (garbanzo beans) or kidney or
  flageolet beans or 1 cup dried
  (see page 143 for cooking time)

2 bulbs (heads) fennel, trimmed and
  cut into wedges from root to tip

Toss into the spicy mixture over a gentle heat. Mix very well.

4 ripe tomatoes, chopped or blended to a pulp or 1 400g (14oz) can tomatoes, whizzed in a blender

Stir into the vegetables, cover and bake in the oven for 35–40 minutes, or until the carrots are soft.

4 tablespoons cider vinegar
handful of fresh chopped chives (optional)

Sprinkle the vinegar over as soon as you take the dish from the oven, cover and leave for 3 minutes. Serve sprinkled with the fresh chopped chives, if using.

Malay-spiced Tofu

Use a large, non-stick pan without a plastic or wooden handle for this recipe. A heavy, enamelled, iron pan is also good.

SERVES 4–6

OVEN: 220°C/425°F/GAS MARK 7

115g (4oz/⅓ cup) fresh root ginger, peeled and grated
15 garlic cloves, peeled
2 fresh or dried red chilli peppers
juice of 1 large lemon

Blend to a paste in a blender or with a pestle and mortar.

500g (1lb 2oz/2 cups) fresh organic tofu, cut into bite-sized pieces
115ml (4fl oz/½ cup) tamari
4 tablespoons cornflour (cornstarch) or arrowroot

Mix gently with half the ginger paste, and leave to marinate (overnight if you can, but allow about 30 minutes if you've made a spontaneous decision to cook this dish).

4 tablespoons cold-pressed oil
4 onions, chopped
6 star anise

Get the oil very hot and fry the onions and star anise together until the onions are good and brown. Stir in the remaining ginger paste and gently add the tofu. Keep the heat high and stir and scrape the pan gently and continually. Place in the oven for 20–25 minutes, scraping and turning gently once during cooking time. Serve with rice or noodles.

Braised Sweet and Sour Carrots

Serve with a stir-fry of vegetables and buckwheat noodles, or try it with Malay-spiced Tofu (page 130) and rice.

Serves 4–6

6 medium carrots, scrubbed and cut into long pieces
3 tablespoons sunflower oil

Sauté together over a high heat until the carrots are just, but only just, browning.

115g (4oz/½ cup) honey

Add to the pan, stir and sizzle well for 4–5 minutes. Reduce the heat, cover and cook very gently for 5 minutes.

140ml (¼ pint/⅔ cup) cider vinegar
4 tablespoons tamari

Remove the lid, increase the heat and stir in the vinegar and tamari. Simmer until the carrots are soft.

2 tablespoons arrowroot or cornflour (cornstarch) or potato flour, mixed to a smooth runny paste with 140ml (¼ pint/⅔ cup) apple juice

Add to the pan and stir well, until thickened and clear.
Check for flavour balance. It may need a spoonful more of honey or vinegar depending on your taste.

Galette of Parsnips and Cashew Nuts

Fresh tarragon makes a good alternative to the parsley.

SERVES 4–6

OVEN: 190°C/375°F/GAS MARK 5

1.5kg (3lb) parsnips, scrubbed and chopped into 1cm (½-inch) slices

Cook in boiling water for 10 minutes.

2 onions, finely chopped
3 tablespoons olive oil
2 teaspoons dried sage
2 teaspoons dried thyme

Soften the onions in a pan with the oil and add the herbs.

455g (1lb/3 cups) whole cashew nuts
2 tablespoons tamari
1 teaspoon black pepper
115g (4oz/2 cups) soft brown breadcrumbs
55g (2oz/1 cup) chopped fresh parsley

Finely chop half the cashews and mix well with everything but the parsnips and parsley. Grease a 20–25cm (8–10-inch) loose-bottomed cake tin or ovenproof dish, spread a layer of whole cashew nuts over the base, then a layer of parsnip slices. It looks good if you stand some round the side too. Spread the breadcrumb mixture over the top and a thick sprinkling of fresh parsley over that. Continue layering the ingredients, ending with parsnips. Cover with foil and bake for 35–40 minutes.

Remove from the oven, let stand for 10 minutes, then turn out onto a warm plate. Slice with a sharp knife and serve with gravy.

Aromatic Glazed Turnips

2 tablespoons honey
2 tablespoons olive oil
3 bay leaves
sprig of fresh thyme (optional)

Melt together in a roasting pan.

approx. 16 baby turnips, trimmed and scrubbed
8 whole shallots or 4 small onions, cut into quarters
115ml (4fl oz/½ cup) water

Add to the pan. Stir to coat the vegetables and bake for about 35 minutes, until the turnips are tender and well browned.

Turn out onto a warmed serving dish and scrape and stir the pan juices, then pour them over the top of the turnips to serve.

Creamed Garlic Potatoes

6–8 medium potatoes, peeled and chopped
6 garlic cloves
285ml (½ pint/ 1 ⅓ cups) soya milk
water to cover

Boil together until the potatoes are tender, then drain. (You can keep the cooking liquid to make a soup.)

4 tablespoons olive oil
grating of nutmeg
pinch of ground black pepper

Add to the cooked potatoes and mash really well. (If you have a mouli you will be able to achieve the ultimate in smoothness.)
Serve as it is or you can pop it in a greased dish and brown in the oven for 10 minutes.

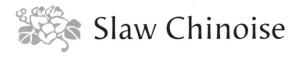

Slaw Chinoise

1 small white cabbage, really finely shredded
115g (4oz/2 cups) shredded Chinese leaves
2 bunches spring onions (scallions), sliced
1 sweet apple, cut into fine strips or grated
55g (2oz/1 cup) mung bean sprouts

Mix together.

2 tablespoons whole almonds
2 tablespoons sesame seeds

Toast gently in a dry pan (keep the lid handy so that the sesame seeds do not jump out all over the cooker). Cool and chop.

2 tablespoons sunflower oil
1 teaspoon roasted sesame oil
2 tablespoons cider vinegar
1 generous teaspoon clear honey
½ teaspoon ground black pepper
2 teaspoons tamari

Blend together and gently mix with the vegetables and toasted nuts.

Vegetable Biriani

5cm (2-inch) stick of cinnamon
6 cloves
4 cardamom pods
1 tablespoon whole cumin seeds
2 bay leaves
6 tablespoons olive oil
3 medium onions, finely grated
5cm (2-inch) piece of fresh root ginger, grated
2 cloves garlic, grated

Heat the whole spices and the bay leaves in the oil until they are just smoking (the bay leaves will blacken). Throw in the other ingredients, stir for a few minutes and enjoy the smell, then reduce the heat. Cover tightly and cook gently for 10 minutes until the onions are soft and slushy.

3 medium potatoes, chopped into even, bite-size pieces
2 medium carrots, cut into small dice
1 small cauliflower, cut into small florets, stems and leaves finely chopped

Stir into the onions over a gentle heat. Replace the lid and cook for 5 minutes.

4 teaspoons tomato purée (tomato paste)
2 teaspoons turmeric
2 teaspoons ground cumin
2 teaspoons ground coriander (cilantro)
juice of ½ lemon
3 tablespoons tamari soy sauce

Stir in a bowl to form a thick, smooth paste. Add to the vegetables, increase the heat and stir and sizzle for 5 minutes until the spices are well mixed and smelling good.

225g (8oz/1⅔ cups) shelled fresh peas and/or broad (fava) beans
225g (8oz/heaping 1 cup) brown basmati rice
water

Stir the peas or beans and rice well into the mix, cover them with water and give the pan a shake. The water should be 2.5cm/1 inch over the top of the mixture. Once boiling, cover tightly and reduce the heat to a very quiet simmer for 40 minutes (or place in a moderate oven at 180°C/350°F/Gas Mark 4 for 45 minutes). The liquid should be fully absorbed and the vegetables soft.

Channa Dhal with Leaves

This dhal is rich and mellow. Try it served with rice or cooked grains. If you want to serve it as a soup, add vegetable stock at the end.

225g (8oz/1 cup) yellow split peas
1.2 litres (2 pints/5 cups) water
1 teaspoon low-salt bouillon powder (optional)
1 teaspoon turmeric

Bring to the boil, reduce the heat to a gentle simmer, then partially cover and cook for 40 minutes until the split peas are soft. Keep the heat gentle as the water boils over easily and can make a real mess of your stove. Remove from the heat and give it a little whisk to break up some of the split peas.

2 tablespoons olive oil
2 bay leaves
1 teaspoon whole black mustard seeds
1 teaspoon whole cumin seeds
short stick of cinnamon
4 whole cloves

Heat the oil in a big heavy pan, add the bay leaves and spices and let them brown (to nearly burnt) and begin to smoke. Be confident here as the smoky taste is very good with split peas.

2.5cm (1-inch) piece of fresh root ginger, grated
340g (12oz/6 cups) fresh spinach or chard leaves, roughly chopped with any tough stems removed

Quickly stir into your smoking pan, adding the ginger first. Watch out for spluttering. Stir to coat with the oil and spices. When the leaves have wilted down, pour in the split peas. The effect can be somewhat volcanic, so be careful and make sure you use a big pan. All this bubbling is worth it as it does combine the flavours wonderfully. Reduce the heat and simmer for 5 minutes to cook the leaves.

juice of 1 big lemon
1 small fresh green chilli pepper, finely chopped (optional)

Sprinkle on top just before serving.

Braised Squash with Green Lentils

120g (4½oz/½ cup) whole green lentils

Cook in water or vegetable stock for 40–45 minutes, until soft.

2 tablespoons olive oil
10 spring onions (scallions), chopped into 2.5cm (1-inch) lengths
2 garlic cloves, peeled and sliced
sprig of fresh thyme
2 bay leaves
1 teaspoon ground black pepper
680g (1½lb/5 cups) yellow-fleshed sweet squash (butternut, red onion or sweet
pumpkin, etc.), cut into bite-size pieces, seeds and fibres removed (if young and
fresh, you shouldn't need to peel it)

Heat the oil and soften the onions and garlic with the herbs and seasoning.
Add the squash. Stir, mix together and cook gently for 6–7 minutes. Add the cooked
lentils and stir in gently.

455g (1lb/2 cups) fresh tomatoes, finely chopped or 395g (14oz) can tomatoes,
finely chopped with juice
1 tablespoon tamari
juice of 1 lemon

Add to the pan and cook very gently for another 20 minutes or so, stirring
occasionally. The dish should be soft and moist, but not runny, so allow some of the
liquid to evaporate.

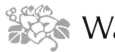

Warm Cauliflower Salad

This dish looks pretty decorated with mint sprigs, a trail of light tahini and a few toasted walnuts.

1 cauliflower, divided into florets, stalk and tiny leaves shredded

Cook in boiling water for 7 minutes, drain and put into a warm serving bowl.

juice of 1 lemon
2 teaspoons cider vinegar
2 tablespoons fresh parsley, chopped
1 tablespoon fresh mint, chopped
1 tablespoon light tahini
1 teaspoon ground black pepper

Whisk together. Pour over the warm cauliflower and serve at once.

Creamy Vegetable Risotto

1 medium onion, finely chopped
115g (4oz/1⅓ cups) firm
   mushrooms, finely chopped
5 tablespoons olive oil

1 large carrot, finely chopped
2 courgettes (zucchini), finely chopped
2 bay leaves
1 tablespoon dried basil

Make sure all the vegetables are cut into tiny pieces. In a heavy pan, sauté everything together gently for a few minutes.

340g (12oz/heaping 1½ cups) brown rice
55g (2oz/⅓ cup) wild rice (optional)
2 tablespoons low-salt bouillon powder
850ml (1½ pints/3¾ cups) water to cover by 2.5cm (1 inch)

Stir the rice into the vegetables and add the bouillon powder and water. Bring to the boil, lower the heat and cover, then simmer until the rice is soft and the liquid absorbed (approximately 35 minutes). Remove from the heat and place a clean cloth or kitchen towel between the pan and the lid to absorb the steam and to fluff up the rice.

55g (2oz/¼ cup) plain
   silken tofu
1 teaspoon ground black pepper

2 tablespoons tamari soy sauce

2 tablespoons soya milk

Whizz together in a blender or food processor until smooth, then stir gently into the rice and heat through.

3 tablespoons nutritional yeast flakes   3 tablespoons fresh parsley, chopped

Tip the rice into a warm serving dish and sprinkle the yeast flakes and parsley on top.

Middle Eastern Bean and Vegetable Casserole

Another one-pot wonder, but not one to try and hurry. Serve in wide, shallow bowls with bread.

225g (8oz/heaping 1 cup) dried beans, such as haricots (navy), cannellini or flageolets

Bring to the boil in a large pan of water, boil for 10 minutes and remove from the heat. Allow to stand for 10 minutes, then drain. Return the beans to the cleaned pan, add 5 cups of water and bring to the boil. Simmer for approximately 1½ hours.

1 large onion, chopped
1 medium carrot, scrubbed or peeled and chopped
4 cloves garlic, sliced
sprigs or sprinklings of fresh or dried thyme, rosemary and oregano

225g (8oz/1⅔ cups) celeriac (celery root), peeled and chopped
5 tomatoes, chopped
handful of fresh parsley, chopped
1 tablespoon low-salt bouillon powder
½ teaspoon ground black pepper
1 teaspoon ground cumin

Add to the beans and their liquid, cover and continue to simmer gently for 45 minutes until the beans are very soft. If you want to go away and do something else, it is best to cook the beans in the oven at 180°C/350°F/Gas Mark 4.

juice of 1 lemon
handful of fresh parsley, roughly chopped

2 tablespoons olive oil (optional)

Stir into the beans, squashing some of them against the side of the pan with a spoon to thicken the juices.

Poppy Seed and Sour Cream Pasta

Delicious with baked or steamed courgettes (zucchini) sprinkled with a little tarragon.

SERVES 4–6

OVEN: 180°C/350°F/GAS MARK 4

225g (8oz/2½ cups) wholemeal (whole-wheat) pasta

Cook in boiling water until tender. Drain.

90ml (3fl oz/⅓ cup) lemon juice
2 tablespoons olive oil
1 tablespoon miso
1 tablespoon tamari
225g (8oz/1 cup) tofu
15g (½oz/⅓ cup) fresh chives, chopped

Blend until smooth in a food processor (if you use a blender, you may need to add a little water to keep it moving).

30g (1oz/¼ cup) poppy seeds
ground black pepper, to taste
pinch of paprika

Stir the poppy seeds into the cream and mix into the pasta.
Turn into a greased, ovenproof dish, sprinkle with some ground black pepper and paprika and bake for about 20 minutes.

Starry Quinoa Pilaff – Persian Style

850ml (1 ½ pints/3¾ cups) water
340g (12oz/2 cups) quinoa

Bring the water to the boil. Add the quinoa, return to the boil, cover and simmer very gently for 15 minutes. Tip into a colander.

140ml (¼ pint/⅔ cup) olive oil
455g (1lb/2½ cups) small, firm okra (ladies fingers), sliced quite thinly
    to form little stars
2 tablespoons tomato purée (tomato paste)
225g (8oz/1 cup) peas
1 medium onion, very finely chopped
3 garlic cloves, thinly sliced
2 tomatoes, finely chopped
2 teaspoons cumin seeds
1 teaspoon ground black pepper

Heat the oil in a large pan (a wok is ideal) over a high heat. Add the okra slices and toss about quickly until just browning. Lower the heat a little, mix in the tomato purée (tomato paste) and fry for a minute or two. Add the other ingredients and keep stirring and tossing together for 5 minutes or so. Lower the heat, cover and cook for 8 minutes more. Uncover, reduce any liquid that is left over a high heat for a couple of minutes and add the quinoa. Mix well. Cover and let stand for 10 minutes.

55g (2oz/1 cup) chopped fresh coriander (cilantro)
2 tablespoons tamari (optional)

Toss into the pilaff as you serve.

Potato and Mushroom Curry

4 tablespoons sunflower oil
1 cinnamon stick
4 whole cloves
2 bay leaves
2 teapoons cumin seeds

Fry together for 2-3 minutes.

2 medium onions, finely chopped
2 x 5cm (2-in) chunks of fresh root ginger, peeled and finely grated
4 garlic cloves, finely grated
1 teapoon tomato purée (tomato paste)
4 tomatoes, chopped

Add to the oil and fry for a few minutes, stirring all the time. Reduce the heat, cover and cook for a further 10 minutes.

2 teaspoons turmeric
2 teapoons ground cumin
2 teaspoons ground coriander

Add to the onions, stir well and fry for 2–3 minutes longer.

4 medium potatoes, cut into approximately 2.5cm (1-in) cubes
350g (12 oz/3 cups) whole button mushrooms

Stir into the pan, making sure that the potatoes are well coated with the spices.

300ml (½ pint/1 cup) water
2 tablespoons tamari

Add to the pan. Stir well, cover and cook over a very low heat for 30 minutes. Stir after 15 minutes and add a little more water if it is beginning to stick. Cook gently until the potatoes are really soft. Serve with rice and a wedge of lemon or raita.

Middle Eastern Rice Salad

340g (12oz/2 cups) cooked brown rice (1 cup uncooked) *(see page 124 for cooking time)*
6 chopped dates, fresh or dried
3 tablespoons toasted cashew nuts
4 spring onions (scallions), finely sliced
2 tablespoons tamari
1 teaspoon toasted fennel seeds
1 teaspoon toasted cumin seeds
juice of 1 juicy lemon
3 tablespoons olive oil

Gently mix together and set to one side to 'develop' for about 30 minutes.

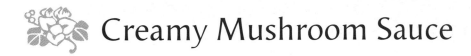

Creamy Mushroom Sauce

3 tablespoons olive oil
225g (8oz/2 cups) mushrooms, finely sliced
2 teaspoons vegetable stock (bouillon) powder or cube
½ teaspoon ground black pepper

Sauté together over a moderate heat until the mushrooms are beginning to soften.

2 level tablespoons unbleached white flour or wholemeal (whole-wheat) flour

Add to the mushrooms and stir well over a gentle heat.

570ml (1 pint/2½ cups) soya milk

Gradually add to the pan, stirring continuously. Increase the heat a little and stir while the sauce thickens.

Cook for another few minutes and serve over tagliatelle or use to layer lasagne and cooked spinach.

Mustard Sauce for Grilled (Broiled) Vegetables

Makes enough to coat a main course of vegetables for two people.

2 tablespoons yellow mustard seeds, soaked overnight in cider vinegar, or
   organic wholegrain mustard
2 tablespoons clear honey
2 tablespoons tamari
1 tablespoon olive oil
ground black pepper, to taste

Whizz together in a blender.

Spoon or spread this sauce on vegetables and grill (broil) for a tasty snack or side dish. Try it on the following, for example:

- halved tomatoes – 10 minutes
- thin slices of aubergine (eggplant) – 10 minutes each side
- thin slices of courgette (zucchini) – 10 minutes each side
- onion wedges – 15 minutes each side
- cooked whole corn cobs – 10 minutes, turning during cooking
- parboiled slices of potato – 5 minutes each side
- parboiled slices of parsnip – 5 minutes each side
- thick slices of fresh tofu – 5 minutes each side

Desserts

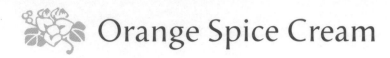

Orange Spice Cream

225–285g (8–10oz / 1 ½ cups) silken tofu
finely grated rind (zest) of 1 large orange
140ml (¼ pint / ⅔ cup) soya milk
1 heaped teaspoon ground mixed spice (apple pie spice)
1 level teaspoon ground cinnamon
2 tablespoons apple juice concentrate or clear honey or date syrup

Whizz in a blender until smooth.

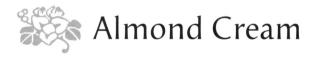

Almond Cream

175g (6oz / 2 cups) ground almonds
300ml (½ pint / 1⅓ cups) soya milk
1 teaspoon almond essence
50g (2oz / ¼ cup) silken tofu (optional)
2 tablespoons apple juice concentrate

Blend until smooth.

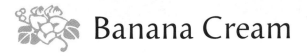

Banana Cream

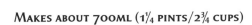

2 bananas
285ml (½ pint/1⅓ cups) soya milk
3 tablespoons cooked brown rice or rice porridge
1 level teaspoon grated nutmeg

Blend until smooth.

Spiced Apple Cake

A moist cake that keeps really well – as long as no-one knows where it is.

455g/1lb sweet apples, grated with skin on
450ml (16fl oz/2 cups) boiling water
285g (10oz/2 cups) raisins
3 tablespoons olive oil
140g (5oz/scant ½ cup) honey
2 tablespoons maple syrup
2 teaspoons ground cinnamon
2 teaspoons ground nutmeg
½ teaspoon ground cloves

Mix together in a large bowl and leave to cool a little.

455g (1lb/heaping 3 cups) wholemeal (whole-wheat) flour
2 teaspoons baking powder

Sift together into the bowl and quickly mix in the fruit mixture. Turn into a greased 25cm/10-inch round cake pan or 1kg/2lb loaf pan and bake in the oven for 1 hour. Test with a skewer – if it comes out a bit sticky, allow another 10-minutes' cooking time. Cool, wrap tightly and store in an airtight container.

Stuffed Baked Apples with Blackberry Sauce

SERVES 4

OVEN: 180°C/350°F/GAS MARK 4

115g (4oz/½ cup) finely ground almonds
2 tablespoons set or clear honey
pinch of cinnamon
4 medium sweet apples, cored (Cox's or Russets are good)

Stir and knead together the almonds, honey and cinnamon to form a thick, 'mouldable' mixture. Form into 4 little sausage shapes and push these down into the cored apples, leaving a little mound on the top of each. Place in a small, greased, ovenproof dish that they fit snugly into, cover and bake for 1½ hours, or until soft but not breaking up.

225g (8oz/1⅓ cups) fresh blackberries
2 tablespoons honey or apple juice concentrate
juice of 1 lemon

While the apples are baking, bring the blackberries, honey or apple juice concentrate and lemon juice to a gentle boil in a heavy-based pan. Cool and push through a strainer to remove the seeds.

Serve the apples hot or chilled on individual plates with a little pool of sauce beside them.

Italian Almond Pudding

Apple with cinnamon and cloves is a classic combination but this recipe also works well with other fruit – such as pears with nutmeg, fresh figs with cinnamon or cherries cooked with a vanilla pod (vanilla bean).

SERVES 4–6

OVEN: 180°C/350°F/GAS MARK 4

455g (1lb) chopped dessert apples
pinch of cinnamon
pinch of ground cloves
2 tablespoons apple juice or water

Cook the apples gently with the spices and apple juice or water until tender.

170g (6oz/1 cup) organic white flour
170 g (6oz/1 cup) wholemeal (whole-wheat) flour
115g (4oz/1 cup) chopped almonds

Sift the flours and mix well with the almonds in a large bowl.

115g (4oz/½ cup) soya margarine
7 tablespoons clear honey
3 teaspoons almond essence

Melt gently together and add to the flour and almonds mixture in the bowl. Stir well. Turn into a deep, ovenproof dish and spread the cooked apples over the top. Bake for approximately 1 hour.

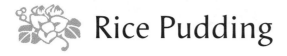

Rice Pudding

This is very good with the addition of a vanilla pod (vanilla bean) or some grated nutmeg or dried fruit.

SERVES 4–6

OVEN: 170°C/325°C/GAS MARK 3

85g (3oz/½ cup) organic brown rice
1 litre (1¾ pints/4½ cups) soya milk

Put together in a heavy-based pan and simmer very gently, covered, for 2 hours. There is no need to stir, but do make sure the heat is very low.

Alternatively, place the ingredients in a greased ovenproof casserole dish and bake, covered, for 2–3 hours. For the best result, though, make the Rice Pudding in a slow cooker, cooking for 4 hours or overnight.

Date and Banana Cookies

MAKES 18–20

OVEN: 200°C/400°F/GAS MARK 6

85g (3oz/½ cup) dried dates, finely chopped
85g (3oz/⅔ cup) walnuts, finely chopped
3 medium bananas, mashed
170g (6oz/2 cups) oats
3 tablespoons olive or cold pressed sunflower oil
1 teaspoon vanilla essence

Mix everything together really well and put tablespoons of the mixture onto an oiled baking sheet. Flatten them down a bit and bake for about 20 minutes, until golden.

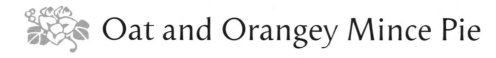

Oat and Orangey Mince Pie

SERVES 4–6

OVEN: 180°C/350°F/GAS MARK 4

85g (3oz/⅓ cup) soya margarine
5 tablespoons olive oil
grated rind (zest) of 1 orange
455g (1lb/3 cups) wholemeal (whole-wheat) flour, sifted
water, to mix

Mix the margarine, oil and orange rind (zest) into the flour, then stir in just enough water for the mixture to come together into a dough (batter). Roll out and use to line a 23cm (8-inch) flan tin.

455g (1lb) organic sugar-free mincemeat or dates or dried fruit of your choice soaked in orange juice

Fill the pastry case with mincemeat or your choice of filling.

115g (4oz/1½ cups) oats
2 tablespoons clear honey
1 tablespoon sunflower or olive oil

Mix together and gently press onto the filling. Bake in the oven for 35–40 minutes.

Poached Pears with Fresh Strawberry Coulis

I hardly need to say that a tofu cream adds extra luxury to this dessert. If you can get some fresh figs, they behave very well when given this treatment too!

4 firm, ripe pears, peeled, cored and halved
300ml (½ pint/1 cup) apple juice concentrate or natural fruit concentrate
    (strawberry or exotic fruit is very good)
600ml (1 pint/2 cups) water

Place the pears flat side down in a deep roasting dish or casserole. Add the liquids, cover and cook gently until the pears are soft – approximately 40 minutes. (Keep the heat low – they don't like to boil madly.) Remove the pears to a serving dish. Boil the juices left in the pan to reduce to about half the volume to form a syrup, and pour over the pears. Chill.

450g (1lb/3 cups) fresh strawberries
juice of 1 lemon
2 tablespoons syrup from the pears

Whizz in a blender until smooth. Serve the pears with a jug of sauce or arrange on individual plates with a little of their syrup and a pool of Fresh Strawberry Coulis.

Drinks

Power-packing Juice Tonic

This delicious energy drink is a good blood builder so it is helpful during your period, if you suffer from anaemia or if you are pregnant. It's also incredibly versatile: it can be served as a salad if you don't put it through the juicer.

MAKES ABOUT 570ML (1 PINT/2½ CUPS)

2 medium fresh beetroot, peeled and grated
3 medium carrots, scrubbed/peeled and grated
2 sweet apples, grated
½ cucumber, thinly sliced
2 tablespoons fresh parsley, chopped
1 tablespoon fresh mint leaves, chopped
juice and zest of a large orange

Combine in a bowl (or juice and drink immediately).

1 teaspoon runny honey (optional)
1 teaspoon walnut oil (optional)
1 teaspoon tamari soy sauce (optional)
½ teaspoon ground black pepper
2 tablespoons toasted walnuts, chopped

Mix and sprinkle over the salad to serve. It's also very good in a sandwich or pitta bread with tahini.

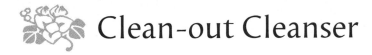

Clean-out Cleanser

½ cucumber, chopped
½ firm cabbage, chopped
2 handfuls of parsley, chopped
sprigs of mint
6 sticks of celery, chopped
2 apples, chopped

Pass through your juicer and enjoy at once.

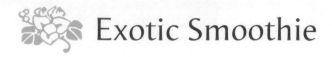

Exotic Smoothie

1 sweet juicy melon, seeds and skin removed and flesh chopped
1 ripe mango, peeled and chopped
2 bananas, peeled and chopped
4 sweet apples, roughly chopped
½ fresh pineapple

Pass through your juicer and enjoy immediately.

Glossary of Medical and Nutritional Terms

allergen	substance promoting an allergic reaction
angina	heart pain caused by lack of oxygen in the heart muscle, normally due to narrowing of the heart's arteries
antioxidant	substance which retards deterioration by oxidation, especially of oils, fats and foods
cancer promoter	increases cancer cell activity once already cancerous
caprilic acid	weak acid used to help acidify the body to prevent the growth of yeasts such as *Candida Albicans*
co-factors	chemicals required to promote the activity of another chemical (e.g. vitamins)
DNA	deoxyribonucleic acid, the main constituent of the chromosomes of all organisms
electrical polarization	presence of an electrical charge gradient
enzymes	proteins produced by living cells which act as catalysts in biochemical reactions such as digestion and metabolism
essential fatty acids	fatty acids which are essential for and are not synthesized by the body
gamma irradiation	irradiation of food with gamma rays, which are electromagnetic rays of shorter wavelength and higher energy than X-rays
hormone-dependent	cancer whose growth is promoted by the presence of hormones
hydrocarbon	any organic compound containing only hydrogen and carbon
hydrogenated fatty acids	fatty acids with an hydroxyl unit attached (i.e. oxygen/hydrogen unit); they are unstable and potentially disruptive to the body
initiator	starts off cancer cell development
kilojoule	measure of energy equal to 1,000 joules
malabsorption	imperfect or defective absorption of nutrients through the gut wall
metabolize	referring to the chemical process which occurs in living organisms resulting in growth, energy production, waste elimination, etc.
oxidative damage	damage to tissues and biochemical processes via free radicals
phytochemical	plant chemical
saltpetre	potassium nitrate, used to preserve meat
transmembrane potential	an electrical charge gradient on two sides of a cell membrane

References

CHAPTER 1

1. Office of Population Censuses & Surveys
2. Chronic Diseases Control Branch, Bal & Forrester, *Cancer* 72 (3 DSuppl): 1005–10
3. Junshi Chen, T. Colin Campbell, Li Junyao and Richard Petto, *A diet lifestyle and mortality in China* (Ithaca, NY: Cornell University Press, 1990)
4. Dr Margaret Thorogood, *British Medical Journal* 308 (28th June 1994): 6945
5. London School of Tropical Hygiene, *British Medical Journal*, June 1994
6. J. Westin, and E. Richter, 'The Israeli Breast Cancer Anomaly', *Annals New York Academy of Sciences*, 609 (1990): 269–79
7. Professor David Orr, c/o The Schumacher Society, Bideford, Devon, UK
8. Bristol Cancer Help Centre Cancer and Nutrition Database, 1993

CHAPTER 3

1. Office of Population Censuses & Surveys

CHAPTER 4

1. (a) W. J. Blot *et al.*, 'Nutrition intervention trials in Linxian (Supplementation with specific vitamin/mineral combinations, cancer incidence and disease specific mortality in the general population)', *Journal National Cancer Institute* 85.18 (September 15, 1993): 1483–92; (b) J. Y. Li *et al.*, 'Nutrition trials in Linxian (Multiole vitamin/mineral supplementation, cancer incidence, and disease-specific mortality among adults with esophageal dysplasia)', *Journal of the National Cancer Institute* 85.18 (September 15, 1993): 1492–98
2. Dr Sandra Goodman, *Nutrition and Cancer: State of the Art* (London: Green Library Publications, 1995)
3. Ferrari, *Biochem. e. Biophys. Acta* 1007 (1989): 3035
4. (a) Dr Rosy Daniel and Dr Sandra Goodman, 'Cancer and Nutrition: The Positive Scientific Evidence', Bristol Cancer Help Centre, July 1994; (b) Nutrition Database, Bristol Cancer Help Centre, July 1993
5. *Lancet* (review article) 347 (January 1996): 249
6. Dr Sandra Goodman, *Vitamin C: The Master Nutrient* (Keats Publishing Inc., 1991)
7. Nutrition Database, Bristol Cancer Help Centre, July 1993

8. Ibid.

9. W. V. Judy, J. H. Hall, W. Dugan, P. D. Toth and Karl Folkers, 'Coenzyme Q10 reduction of adriamycin cardio-toxicity', in Karl Folkers and Y. Yamamura (eds), *Biochemical and Clinical Aspects of Coenzyme Q10*, vol.4 (Amsterdam: Elsevier, 1984)

10. Nutrition Database, Bristol Cancer Help Centre, July 1993; Michael Lerner, Choices in Healing (Cambridge, MA: MIT Press): 234, 235

11. Lockwood, Moesgaard, Hanioka and Folkers, 'Partial and complete regression of breast cancer in patients in relation to dosage of coenzyme Q10, antioxidant vitamins and fatty acids', *Biochemical & Biophysical Research Communication* March 30th, 1994

Bibliography and Further Reading

Scientific

Daniel, Dr Rosy and Goodman, Dr Sandra, 'Cancer and Nutrition: The Positive Scientific Evidence' (Bristol Cancer Help Centre, 1994)

Flytlie, Dr Knut and Madsen, Bjorn F, 'Q10 – Body Fuel: The natural way to a healthier body – and a longer life' (Denmark: Norhaven rotation A/S)

Goodman, Dr Sandra, *Vitamin C: The Master Nutrient* (Keats Publishing, 1991)

Goodman, Dr Sandra, *Nutrition and Cancer: State of the Art* (Green Library Publications, 1995)

NUTRITION

Holford, Patrick, *The Optimum Nutrition Bible* (Santa Cruz, CA: Crossing Press, 1999)

Holford, Patrick, *Say No to Cancer* (London: Piatkus, 1999)

Olivier, Suzannah, *The Breast Cancer Prevention and Recovery Diet* (London: Penguin, 2000)

Olivier, Suzannah, *The Detox Manual* (New York: Simon and Schuster, 2001)

Plant, Jane, PhD, *Your Life in your Hands: Understanding, Preventing and Overcoming Breast Cancer* (New York: St Martin's Press, 2000)

COOKERY

Elliot, Rose, *The Bean Book* (London: Thorsons, 2000)

Elliot, Rose, *Not Just a Load of Old Lentils* (London: Thorsons, 1994)

Gavin, Paola, *Italian Vegetarian Cooking* (Little, Brown, 1991)

Hom, Ken, *Ken Hom's Vegetarian Cookery* (London: BBC Books, 1995) (Chinese Cookery)

Jaffrey, Madhur, *Eastern Vegetarian Cooking* (London: Jonathan Cape, 1983)

Jaffrey, Madhur, *Indian Cookery* (London: BBC Books, 1996) (not exclusively vegetarian)

Kenton, Leslie, *Raw Energy Recipes* (London: Ebury, 1994)

Leneman, Leah, *Early Vegan* Cooking (London: Thorsons, 1998)

Ross, Janet, *Leaves from Our Tuscan Kitchen* (London: Penguin, 1997)

Sen, Jane, *The Healing Foods Cookbook* (London: Thorsons, 2000)

Sen, Jane, *More Healing Foods* (London: Thorsons, 2001)

Wakeman, Alan, *The Vegan Cookbook* (London: Faber & Faber, 1986)

Although *Indian Cookery* is not a vegetarian cookery book, and the two Italian books are not vegan, they do contain many vegan recipes to give you inspiration. Nowadays if you look in the cookery section of any good bookshop you will find many vegetarian and vegan cookery books, and the BBC publishes a vegetarian cooking-guide supplement each month.

Index

Healing Foods Cookbook
THE VEGAN WAY TO WELLNESS

Jane Sen

Using really fresh, whole ingredients to create an inspired range of ultra-simple, exciting new dishes, Jane Sen's sensational-tasting recipes are so good for you that you'll be able to enjoy them in the knowledge that your body is saying 'thank you'.

'Exciting and unusual flavours – delicious enough to fob off teenagers and children without them suspecting they are eating healthily. She writes with a sense of fun I don't remember finding in more leaden wholefood books. I recommend it.'

DEIRDRE MCQUILLAN, SUNDAY TELEGRAPH

'The *Healing Foods Cookbook* contains low-fat recipes rich in the nutrients you need to fight cancer. Find out how you can change your diet – it could save your life.'

MARTHA ROBERTS, SUN

More Healing Foods
OVER 100 DELICIOUS RECIPES TO INSPIRE HEALTH AND WELLBEING

Jane Sen

The follow-up to Jane Sen's bestselling *Healing Foods Cookbook* is as delicious as healthy eating gets. Her enthusiasm for cookery and simple delight in the ingredients is refreshing in a world where healthy eating all too often means foregoing the enjoyment of food.

These taste-filled, high-nutrition recipes, each free from meat, dairy and added salt or sugar, will boost your health and do you good, especially if your concerns include:

Weight loss · Digestive problems · Heart disease · Cancer · Diabetes · Lack of energy · Fertility problems · Menopause

'Sen's work, which revolves around a vegan low-fat, -salt and -sugar diet has been recognized by heart disease charities for its contribution to healthy eating, and has inspired many cancer patients.'

SONIA PURNELL, GUARDIAN

Make
www.thorsonselement.com
your online sanctuary

www.thorsonselement.com

Get online information, inspiration and
guidance to help you on the path to physical
and spiritual well-being. Drawing on the integrity
and vision of our authors and titles, and with
health advice, articles, astrology, tarot, a
meditation zone, author interviews and events
listings, www.thorsonselement.com is a great
alternative to help create space and peace
in our lives.

So if you've always wondered about practising
yoga, following an allergy-free diet, using the
tarot or getting a life coach, we can point you
in the right direction.

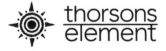

thorsons
element